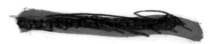

Computerizing Your Medical Office

Computerizing Your Medical Office A Guide for Physicians and Their Staffs
Second Edition

Dot Sellars, CMA-A, COAP

Medical Economics Books
Oradell, New Jersey 07649

Library of Congress Cataloging in Publication Data

Sellars, Dot.
  Computerizing your medical office. Second Edition

  Includes index.
  1. Medicine—Data processing.   2. Medical offices
—Data processing.   3. Microcomputers.   I. Title.
[DNLM: 1. Computers.   2. Office management.   3. Economics,
Medical.   W 80 S467c]
R858.S445   1983   651'.961'02854   83-13487
ISBN 0-87489-480-8

Medical Economics Company Inc.
Oradell, New Jersey 07649

Printed in the United States of America

To the doctors of Insight Physicians, P.C. of Richmond, Virginia and to the many other physicians who have supported me in my educational endeavors and who have encouraged me to share my knowledge; to the educators who have assisted me and who must prepare their students to approach computerization of the medical office in a knowledgeable way; and to the American Association of Medical Assistants, Medical Group Management Association, and Office Automation Society International for giving me the opportunity to stay current with the changes affecting business and medicine.

Contents

Preface

Over the past 5 years, there have been major changes in the health care industry, primarily to decrease the cost of healthcare. Many physicians in private practice, however, have seen their expenses increase and their revenue decrease as a result of these changes. Physicians have had to hire additional personnel—keeping up with precertification and recertification of hospital patients, for example, can be a full time job. Capitation and/or discounted fee-for-service has decreased revenue but increased recordkeeping expenses. It is readily apparent that physicians—or someone representing their interests—must know how the health care changes are affecting the business side of medicine.

Consumer demands for the best possible medical care have contributed to the increased cost of providing that care. Since medical insurance is provided as a fringe benefit by most employers for their employees, third-party payers have continually had to increase their rates. Employers are now looking for ways to decrease the cost of providing health-care benefits for their employees, and third-party payers are offering alternative plans. Employers also are negotiating special provisions in the plans they select.

Gone are the days when one could maintain files by insurance carrier only. In many cases now, maintaining insurance files by carriers *and* employers is mandatory. Health-care programs require varying deductible amounts to be met by the patient prior to any payment from the plan. After the deductible has been met, the plan may also require the patient to pay a co-payment for each visit, and the amount may vary greatly between carriers and between plans. In addition, the contract may require hospital admissions to be approved in advance with a fixed number of days allowed for the condition or treatment. A second surgical opinion may also be required. Preadmission testing may be necessary, and it may also be necessary to perform surgery on the same day as hospital admission. Failure on the part of the physician to abide by these rules may result in payment denial of the claim or payment at 50 percent of the allowable charge. All of these policies and procedures are further complicated by specific billing instructions.

The approval of hospital admission is not a guarantee of insurance coverage. It does not waive any policy provisions that may affect the coverage. You could receive hospital approval for a patient, based upon diagnosis and treatment, even if the patient does not have insurance protection.

Living in an area (Richmond, Virginia) that is a test site center for health maintenance organizations (HMOs), preferred provider organizations (PPOs), and individual practice associations (IPAs) has been an eventful experience. Because a claim can be denied for any reason, there is simply no room for error. Treatment must be authorized, and all instructions followed. The diagnosis must be relevant to the procedure performed. Claims also can be denied for untimely filing (for example, not filed within 90 days of the service rendered, not filed within a specified number of days at the close of the calendar year, not filed within a year, and so on).

Most insurance policies have varying deductible amounts that must be satisfied or paid by the patient prior to any payment by the plan. Co-payments from the patient also will vary. One should know the amount, and for office visits, it should be collected at the time the service is rendered. Another complicating factor is that the charge for procedures performed may vary according to the contractual discounted fee-for-service. Capitation, however, pays a fixed amount for all patients assigned, but it is necessary to maintain records of the procedures performed by patient. Sound complicated? It is!

Outside audits can be performed in many areas, such as medical record documentation, billing procedures, signature on file for release of information and authorization for payment to the physician, codes used for diagnoses and procedures, and so on. Quality assurance is measured by performance standards, and accuracy is a critical factor.

Although HMOs are not yet popular in many areas, they are rapidly overtaking insurance plans. HMOs are designed to control healthcare costs causing major changes in the health-care industry. As a result, many problems may occur in the traditional medical office. Cash flow may be poor, accounts receivable may be high, and there may be a need to implement new systems. Certainly, the effectiveness and efficiency of the medical office needs to be analyzed in an effort to decrease costs and increase earnings. If changes are not made from within, the operating efficiency cannot be improved.

Since machines speed up the work process, a computer system is almost mandatory for managing the business of the medical practice. Advanced technology not only provides better work and increased efficiency but also better internal control. Computer systems do not last forever, however, particularly in the midst of major changes. If you have computerized your business operations in the past, is the system operating at its peak efficiency to serve your current needs? Have you received any program enhancements? A careful analysis of your own individual needs and priorities is essential before choosing a system or changing a system.

Combining the methods of business with the ethics of professionalism can be a challenge, but it is essential for the success of the practice. The art of practicing medicine can suffer from poorly administered professional practice management. A computer system can enhance your business operations if properly planned for and implemented. It is designed to perform the accounting functions, improve cash flow, reduce paperwork, and provide statistical reports for making better decisions.

Acknowledgements

The author wishes to acknowledge the support and encouragement of her family, friends and associates. I thank my publisher for giving me motivational support and assistance—the necessary ingredients for completing the book. I am deeply grateful to Applied Digital Data Systems, Inc. of Hauppauge, New York, Freeman & Morgan Architects, P.C. and Neurosurgical Associates, P.C. of Richmond, Virginia for providing the photographs, forms and/or sketches used in this book.

I. Do You Really Need a Computer?

1. Ten Warning Signs That Could Point You Toward a Computer

Computers have touched the lives of all of us in recent years. Your credit card statements are handled by computer, a number of functions in many cars are performed by microcomputers, a computerized scanner system rings up your groceries at the supermarket, and you may have bought your children a Nintendo or Atari video game system.

More important, you've seen computerization come to the medical profession. Your local independent laboratory utilizes computers, as do the hospitals where you have staff privileges. And, of course, you probably know many colleagues who have already computerized their office operations.

But you haven't done so—yet—even though some of your colleagues with computers have touted the wonders of their new machines. You may think something like, "I've gotten along pretty well without computers up to now. But can I continue to practice good medicine without one?"

This isn't a simple question, and it's one that should be mulled over carefully. I've seen too many physicians rush out to get a computer system simply because a colleague has one. Invariably, physicians who've played this high-technology version of keeping up with the Joneses end up with a system that doesn't really serve their needs.

You don't get a computer just to stay current with the times. A computer will not solve unknown or unspecified problems. What a computer *can* do is make your practice more efficient. An electronic, computer-based system has the advantages of speed, accuracy, and flexibility over manual systems. A computer can store large amounts of information in a small space and can give you quick access to it. It can reduce the need for filing records by hand. And it can store and process the data that are generated when payments are recorded, charges are added, and the like.

If you purchased your computer system more than 5 years ago, no doubt it is still working. At least, it handles your accounts receivable and kicks out insurance claims and statements. But what enhancements have you made to the program to accommodate the changes in billing procedures? An evaluation may reveal that there is manual intervention by your staff.

Does your system allow you to store the patient's co-payment, multiple diagnoses, the amount allowed for payment by the plan, the accident date, etc.? Does it provide storage for special provisions in the insurance contract, such as precert for hospital admission or second surgical opinion required? Does it print the insurance carrier's address on the claim form? Are you confined to only a write-off without the ability to define the write-off? For example, by insurance plan (Blue Cross, Medicare, Medicaid, etc.) do you know how much your write-offs were last year—the difference between allowed and non-allowed charges—caused by your participation in the various plans to abide by the allowed charge as the billable charge?

HMOs also may deduct risk factor fees, and you need to know the amount by each plan. It is conceivable that a percentage of your risk factor fees may be returned to you at the end of the year if the carrier has had a successful year.

Discounted fee-for-service may require the storage for more than one fee schedule. Does your system allow you to do this?

Capitation is complexed—a fixed amount paid to you for a specified number of patients. Procedures must be billed for, as with any patient, but capitation pays you for all the patients assigned to you. Your accounts receivable may be exceedingly high—and false—if your accounting method includes posting payment to each patient's account. You may find large balances on some accounts (which are not collectible) and credit balances on many others, generating an accounts receivable that is not accurate or out of control. How is this situation being handled in your office? Is it on the computer or controlled manually? Have you hired extra help because of it?

Your Office Efficiency

Whether you need a computer to perform these and other functions is what you'll have to decide. Your personal and professional success depends to a large extent on the efficiency of your office. If your staff is still doing things the way things were done 5 years ago, your office is probably not operating at peak efficiency. And if you also have obsolete, inadequate, or unsuitable equipment, you can almost be assured that your office isn't being run in an efficient or cost-effective manner.

Some definite signals will tell you whether your office needs revamping. If any of the following alarms have sounded, it's probably time for you to look into the possibility—and the feasibility—of computerizing your office.

1. Your practice is growing.
2. There are delays in processing insurance claims.
3. Collections have fallen off.
4. Billing schedules are not being met.
5. Your medical assistants have so much paperwork that they don't have time to assist in the delivery of clinical services.
6. Expenses are accelerating.
7. You practice—and need information—at more than one office location.
8. Status information for decision making is sometimes missing.
9. Filing cabinets are taking over your business office.
10. You lack critical information about the type of patients serviced.

Some of these areas may be more important to you than others. But even if only one of these categories applies, your practice may not be operating as efficiently and effectively as it should. And the odds are that if there are problems with your practice, several of these categories will apply.

Just stating the problem areas may not be enough, however, to bring home their importance. Let's look into them in more detail and examine some of the symptoms, too.

1. YOUR PRACTICE IS GROWING. Good business principles stress continuing growth to help ensure success. Planning is a key element in attaining potential growth. In your medical practice, changing office procedures to meet the needs of the community you serve and extending more services to your patients are measures that are usually indicative of the desire to grow. You may have taken on a partner and hired more office personnel in response to growth—or in anticipation of it if you sense a potential increase in patient load. And obviously, an ever-increasing patient load should bring in an ever-increasing stream of revenue.

The potential for growth of your practice means nothing, however, if concrete plans to help ensure that growth have not been made or are not being measured for effectiveness. A computer system will not make your practice grow. But if your practice is already growing—or you expect that it soon will be—it may be time to at least investigate what a computer system can do for you and your practice.

A computer can help you evaluate your community's medical needs and your practice's patient mix. It can be employed to project your personnel needs, assess growth, and analyze income. It can help you conform to practicing as a group, rather than practicing as multiple solo practices within a group.

2. INSURANCE WORK IS A BURDEN. Completing insurance claim forms on behalf of your patients can become burdensome because usually there simply is not enough time to keep up with this task. Although insurance claims are usually received daily, chances are that your office personnel can't complete the forms on a daily basis. In most medical offices, the demands of the patients who are currently receiving services—and the immediate needs of the doctors—lay first claim to the staff's attention. It becomes increasingly difficult to accomplish all the necessary paperwork.

Prioritizing work is essential when a variety of duties must be done. To prioritize, you and your staff list "must do," "should do," and "nice to do" tasks—or something in between. The "must do" jobs get done, but the others may be repeatedly put off until "tomorrow" or until you're out of town or away from the office. Offices like this have no systematic approach to processing claims. Difficult claims are placed at the bottom of the pile. The medical assistant asks herself, "Why should I take 30 minutes to process this difficult claim when I can do three easier ones in the same time?" Understandably, there are many offices—and many medical assistants—operating in this manner.

Some physicians—you may be among them—have tried to deal with the insurance-form problem by putting the burden of claim processing on patients, and charging for the completion of forms that patients can't, or won't, process themselves. Patients, however, are likely to find this job just as annoying and difficult as medical-office personnel do. As the competition for patients continues to heat up, offering to process patients' insurance claims may become an increasingly significant practice builder.

But if you do handle claims routinely, your office should control all claims processing and should not depend on the patient to furnish the "correct" form to file with the insurance carrier. In the past, the diagnoses and/or treatment often determined the necessity for filing an insurance claim, but today most insurance contracts allow for varying deductible amounts to be satisfied or paid by the patient prior to any payment by the plan. Consequently, it is essential for all visits to be filed with the carrier. Is this being accomplished in your office? Do you have a backlog of claims to be filed? What is the turnaround time between receiving the claim form and mailing the completed form to the insurance company? Do you depend on patients to furnish you with forms? Are *you* satisfied with your present insurance claim system? Are your patients satisfied—or are your telephone lines busy with patients inquiring about the status of their insurance claims?

A good insurance-claim-processing system requires a specific method for doing the job in a timely manner. This not only eliminates many telephone calls from and to patients but also eliminates claim processing according to "telephone pressure"—the patient who screams loudest getting his claim processed first.

3. COLLECTIONS HAVE FALLEN OFF. If your collections are less this month than they were last month or are less than the same month's total a year ago, you'd better find out why. For example, if you earned less money this year than last, you may shrug your shoulders and say, "It's just the economy," or "My expenses are greater because of inflation." But it may be more complex than that. A decrease in collections and/or cash flow for one month may not mean anything. But if it starts to become a pattern, you may discover that you're not really in control of the business side of your practice.

Cash flow planning is making sure enough cash is available to operate the practice efficiently during a given period. Operating expenses should be paid regularly and on time. Whenever the cash flow falls off, there should be cause for concern.

Appointment scheduling, insurance claim processing, billing—even the music played in your waiting room—can affect collections and your cash flow. A dissatisfied patient may purposely make you wait for your money. Collecting cash at the time service is rendered is one way of helping to solve a cash flow problem. But remember that you can only *ask*—you can't demand—time-of-service payment. And once the patient leaves the office, he is the one who'll determine what priority your bill will have.

Good business practices and procedures must be employed to maximize income. In many areas of the country, collecting cash at the time service is rendered means collecting the co-payment from the patient. The co-payment may vary from $1 to 50 percent of the *allowed charge* after the deductible amount has been satisfied. We are living in a world of third-party payers, and physicians must abide by all the contracts. To do otherwise would probably kill the practice. As a direct result, cash flow can only be increased by good business practices and procedures. Do you use performance standard as a management tool for measuring the accuracy of billing procedures? Do you have a systematic follow-up system for your accounts receivable, or do you only skim the cream from the top?

4. BILLING SCHEDULES ARE NOT BEING MET. Nobody needs to tell you that physicians are often the last to be paid. After all, most people don't plan for medical expenses in their budgets. They don't plan to be injured or sick, so naturally they don't plan to spend any money on medical care, including their co-payment. A hospital admission or surgery could result in the patient's owing you a large sum of money as their cost-share for services rendered.

Statements need to be rendered on a regular basis; that is, at a set time every month. Billing is a dreaded chore in many offices. The statements are prepared and then left until someone has the time to stuff the envelopes and prepare the mailing. It is done whenever the staff can get to it. Statements may be mailed on the 10th one month and on the 20th the next. What difference does it make? The patients realize that their statements arrive erratically; they figure that if the doctor's in no hurry to collect, why should they be in a hurry to pay? Patients will thus pay their more pressing bills on payday and let the doctor wait a little longer for his money.

Obviously, collections suffer when billing schedules are not met. Bills must be rendered at regular intervals. Just think about your own personal bills: You get the mortgage bill, the credit card bill, the utility company bill, ad infinitum, at about the same time every month. It's almost a reflex on your part to write the checks for these bills. But if you didn't get a bill—or if it didn't come on a fairly rigorous schedule—would you be as quick to reach for your checkbook?

5. PAPERWORK TIES DOWN YOUR OFFICE STAFF. Paperwork is voluminous in most medical offices because it's necessary to provide documentation for just about everything that occurs there. To do otherwise might lead to liability or problems with malpractice suits—or simply to less-than-adequate medical care. For example, if a patient cancels an appointment, it should be so recorded both on his chart and in the appointment book. The turnaround time for answering a life insurance questionnaire should be no longer than about two weeks. Referring physicians must be kept up to date regarding the status of their patients. And third-party payers must be kept informed about patients' treatments and conditions. Records must be maintained for preadmission testing and/or precertification of scheduled hospital admissions as well as recertification of hospital patients, if you feel a longer hospital stay is necessary. And don't forget that if you miss obtaining that second or third surgical opinion, you may not get paid for performing the surgery or paid at 50 percent of the allowed charge. Verification of where the surgery can be performed—inpatient or outpatient—also may be necessary.

Paperwork never stops. The assistants who used to give you a hand in the delivery of clinical services may now be devoting most of their time to paperwork. You may have reached the point where you need additional staff to help you deliver first-rate health-care services. Then again, you may be able to put your current assistants back in the examining and treatment areas—and let the computer handle much of the "paperwork."

6. EXPENSES ARE ACCELERATING. Have your operating expenses been rising rapidly? Have you hired additional staff over the past year—or do you still need more staff—to keep on top of all the necessary work of your office? A careful analysis of your operating costs over the past few years should reveal where the greatest increases in expenditures have occurred. You'll no doubt find that salaries and fringe benefits have added the most to your costs. And if your practice is going to grow, you'll probably need even more personnel to assist you.

But even if you want to add more staff, do you have the space for them? Maybe you'd have to move to larger quarters. Many times, this is an unappealing option. Patients are familiar with your present location and some may not follow you if you move. Your current rent is probably based on a long-term lease and undoubtedly you'll pay much more if you have to find new quarters. Then, too, your new location may not be as convenient for you—to your hospitals, your home, or a second office.

The solution could be a computer. It may eliminate the need for additional personnel. It should also eliminate some expenses that have been increasing in recent years. For example, a report issued by the Dartnell Institute of Business Research revealed that between 1968 and 1980, the cost of writing and mailing an ordinary business letter rose from $2.54 to $6.07. It naturally follows that the cost of writing collection letters for delinquent patients' accounts also had to increase. And for collection letters to serve any useful purpose, they must be sent out regularly—not just when someone in your office has a few minutes available to work on them. Repetitious work such as this, however, is something that can be done well and inexpensively by an office computer system. Add the inflation factor from 1980 to the present time and you'll get today's cost— another significant increase.

Another example: Postage rates are continuing to rise. But if you're sending out, say 200 indentical pieces of mail at once—such as when billing accounts—you may be eligible for special discount rates for bulk mail. If you're not currnetly taking advantage of this saving, you may be able to obtain it as one of the benefits of the computer system. A computer can help you meet the necessary requirements to use first-class presort mail with a minimum of help from office personnel.

7. YOU PRACTICE IN MORE THAN ONE LOCATION. In recent years, there's been a trend for physicians—both solo doctors and groups—to practice in multiple locations. A satellite office may be used strictly for the convenience of seeing patients, while the financial records and all necessary paperwork are handled at the primary office.

Quite often, however, it isn't enough to have just medical records available at a satellite office. Patients may want to pay their bills at time of service but need some additional information from you, so you may need financial information at your fingertips. If this and other information isn't readily available, it's certainly going to hinder both you and your satellite office staff.

Of course, you could take ledger cards to the satellite offices with you. But then you're just asking for trouble. A ledger card should be removed from the file only long enough to make a copy of it. Then, too, you could make copies of all the ledger cards you'll need. But this is an expensive and time-consuming operation. Think about how much easier it would be to punch a few buttons on a video display terminal and instantly have all the necessary information!

8. STATUS INFORMATION IS MISSING. Do you have all the information necessary for making decisions wisely when you need it? Or do you sometimes lack critical information that would be valuable to you in making sound business decisions?

Remember that your accounting system is an information system. It should always be able to provide you with accurate, up-to-date information about your practice when you need it. If, for example, you think that you probably need another assistant to give allergy injections, can you justify it based on accurate, current data? The right information will help you decide whether you need a full-time or a part-time person—or anyone at all. You need to know how many patients are currently receiving allergy injections, and the revenue generated from this specific service, before you can decide whether to increase your overhead in this area. You should also be able to project approximately how much you can expect to generate from these allergy injections if the new assistant is utilized fully. And if the information shows that there's really a need for only a part-time person in this area, you can decide from other information whether she could also be used to perform other office functions if you did, in fact, hire her on a full-time basis.

Ferreting out this information from a manual accounting system isn't impossible, but it's difficult. With the right computer system, the search would be quick and effortless.

Business decisions should not be made by whim or fancy. Missing information can be detrimental to your practice. If you don't have the facts, you probably won't be able to make the most knowledgeable decisions.

9. FILING CABINETS ARE TAKING OVER YOUR BUSINESS OFFICE. Floor space is expensive. Taking up space with bulky filing cabinets holding all your necessary records is a problem that could sharply hinder your office efficiency and productivity. And when an office assistant has to go to two or three different places to look for something, she's not utilizing her time as well as she might be.

Don't get carried away with the idea that a computer can replace files. It can't. But with a computer, you may be able to move files to a storage or less-busy area, out of the bustle of your front desk or business office. (Dividend: A computer and its CRT—cathode-ray tube, or video display screen—looks so much neater than several tiers of filing cabinets with office staffers swerving hard to avoid the sharp corners.)

10. YOUR PRACTICE LACKS DEMOGRAPHIC INFORMATION. Detailed information about your practice and your patients can be very beneficial. Knowing the types of patients you treat can aid you in making better decisions about your practice. For example, do you know how many patients you've treated this month for hypertension? Or how about the percentage of your patients who have medical insurance? If you accept Medicare, do you know how much revenue you receive from it? Do you know the number of appendectomies and mastectomies you've performed, or how many fractures you've treated, in the past three months? Do you know the revenue breakdown for the various procedures that you perform? These are just a few examples of how a computer system could help you. With a computer, this type of data should always be available and easily retrievable.

Where a Computer Might Help You

You've just reviewed 10 possible problems. Several could be due to an inefficient bookkeeping system—a problem many physicians face. Yet the right computer system can give you the mechanism for sound financial management that you may not have with your present system.

Bookkeeping—the Obvious Area

To understand how a computer system might help you more than your current system, first take a quick look at the three types of bookkeeping systems used in physicians' offices: manual, mechanical, and computerized.

MANUAL. There are three varieties of manual systems:

Single-entry. The simplest manual system is known as the single-entry system. Income and expenses are recorded daily but not totaled until the end of the month. Income can be verified by deposit slips, and expenses by canceled checks. Charges are often recorded from the appointment book. The practice checkbook serves as the cash disbursement journal, and the accounts receivable ledger may be the ledger card file. While the single-entry system is easy to use and requires little staff training, it has no built-in financial controls or checks and balances to help prevent mistakes.

Double-entry. The double-entry manual system offers more protection against error because for every transaction, two effects are recorded. If a patient pays $100 on his account, it increases revenue while decreasing accounts receivable. But this system is time-consuming and often requires the skills of a trained bookkeeper.

Pegboard. A third manual system in use today is the pegboard system. To post a payment to the patient's account, the assistant pulls the patient's ledger card and places it on the journal, or daysheet, to record a cash receipt and a decrease in accounts receivable. Only one entry needs to be written—carbon paper or NCR paper takes care of the other entries. This system is still time-consuming and may still lead to errors if the posting isn't done in the presence of the patient.

MECHANICAL. There are, of course, bookkeeping machines, which are somewhat better than most of the manual systems. But with these semiautomated systems, each transaction must be analyzed as to its effect on various accounts before it is entered into the system.

Even the best manual or mechanical bookkeeping system is time-consuming. And while the degree of control varies, each system is subject to human error.

COMPUTERIZED. A computer-based system offers the big advantage of speed as well as additional control, since all financial computations—where many human errors often occur—are performed electronically. With a computer, you can store a large amount of information in a small space—and find it quickly when you need it. The stored information can be automatically brought to a video screen right in front of you or one of your assistants. If a permanent copy is desired, you just need to send a simple command to the printer. And since the computer can process information so quickly, all you'll have to do to get any current figures is push a couple of buttons.

Other Areas for Review

Bookkeeping is only one major area where your practice may need improvement. Only a thorough review of your office practices and procedures can determine how efficiently your office is being run. Often such a study reveals facts that are difficult to accept, because the problems uncovered stem from the lack of a sound management system. Remember, though, that problems must be identified before they can be eliminated—and before the right system can be instituted for the proper delegation of office responsibilities.

The review and evaluation of your office and business practices can be done by you and/or your associates. You may feel more comfortable, however, with having an outside professional—such as a practice management consultant—perform this task. But no matter who does it, any such study should focus on: (1) staff responsibilities, (2) work flow patterns, (3) office space utilization, (4) document preparation, and (5) financial stability. If an in-depth study reveals deficiencies in any of these areas, your practice probably needs some shoring up.

You're not running an efficient practice if you're not making the best use of your time. And if you're not making the best use of your time, your productivity isn't as high as it should be.

Increasing your efficiency will increase your productivity—the dollar amount for services rendered, which, of course, translates into gross income. When a patient is charged for an office visit, for example, it's considered part of a doctor's productivity record. But when the patient actually pays for the office visit, it affects the gross income record. And the higher your gross income, the greater your potential for high net income.

Notice I said *potential*. Just increasing your gross income won't necessarily mean more dollars in your pocket. If your overhead costs are too high, many of the extra dollars you generate through increased productivity will be eaten up by unnecessary expenses. The bottom line, then, is to increase productivity while keeping costs down.

Of course, the primary objective of most physicians is to provide quality patient care. All practices and procedures for the medical office should enhance that quality. Patient care encompasses not just the medical services rendered, but the entire treatment of the patient. It's not a contradiction in terms for a physician to give his patients the best possible care *and* maximize his productivity. The efficient and organized physician will receive high marks both from his patients and from his accountant.

2. What Computerization Can Do for You

One of the few things the average computer cannot tell you is whether or not you need one. What can? The noises your practice makes.

Sound financial management is the key to a successful medical practice. Financial records are vital. The better the information provided by your bookkeeping system, the better you can satisfy your tax and legal requirements, determine your economic progress, and provide a sound basis for financial decision making. So a thorough audit of all your areas of operation should precede any decision about acquiring a computer.

The list in Table 2-1 shows some of the tasks that in-house computer systems are actually performing in medical practices of all sizes. Both business and clinical uses are listed. It's true that such items as in-office CME programs and phone-line hookups to national data banks are the "sizzle" that often attracts physicians to computers. But most experts agree that meat-and-potatoes financial uses come first when considering computer installation.

It is important to realize that no one current computer system handles *all* the items listed. The specific needs and priorities of your own office must be carefully analyzed to determine how a computer could help you most. Ready-made software packages will not necessarily provide all related functions noted in the discussions that follow. Some func-

Table 2-1. *52 Uses for an In-house Computer*

Here are some of the uses doctors in solo, small, and medium-sized practices have found for their in-house systems.

Billing, collecting, and insurance
Accounts receivable
Aging analysis of accounts receivable
Collection letters
Disability and workers' comp claim processing
Disk-to-disk claim processing
Insurance claim processing
Multipurpose billing forms
Patient billing

Accounting
Accounts payable
Annual statements to patients
Cash report
Check register
Check-writing
Cross-posting in multiphysician practices
Daysheet
Deposit slip
Family accounting
General ledger
Income and expense statement
Payroll
Profit and loss statements
Retirement plan accounting
W-2 forms

Practice management
Employee vacation and sick-time records
Hospital lists and charges
Interface with satellite offices
Inventories of drugs and supplies

Practice management (*cont.*)
Ordering drugs and supplies
Patient profiles by age, diagnosis, etc.
Practice profiles by diagnosis, procedure, services
Production reports by physicians
Referral profiles

Scheduling and follow-up
Appointment scheduling
Follow-up scheduling
Patient recall lists
Patient reminders

Clinical
Access to national data banks
CME (continuing medical education) programs
Drug interaction and allergy checks
Literature retrieval
Medical records
Patient education
Prescription-writing
Protocols, diagnosis, and treatment
Research

Word processing
Articles
Consultation reports
Correspondence
Interoffice memos
Labels and addressing
Thank-you letters
Welcome-to-practice letters

tions may need to be customized for your own practice, at greater expense than would be incurred in purchasing a ready-made system.

Also be aware that minicomputers were initially developed as lower-cost alternatives to mainframes. Minis provide extensive communication capabilities and excellent flexibility. Minicomputer software usually is designed for business management functions. Some personal computers (PCs) are not appropriate for the applications discussed here; they are simply not powerful enough and do not possess sufficient memory. PCs use different microprocessors (chips) to provide the varying degree of computing power required.

In response to consumer demand, personal computer hardware has improved significantly. Almost as quickly as new microprocessors are introduced, pressure begins to build for the development of more powerful microprocessors. The user's demand for multitasking operations and multiuser capabilities are examples of the pressure exerted on the manufacturers. The introduction of the 32 bit microprocessor is an example of technological advance resulting from consumer demand. The distinctions noted between the different classes of computers are becoming more difficult to define. The major obstacle at the present time is that the development of operating-system and application software needed to take advantage of the PC hardware capabilities has lagged.

Also be aware that home computers (microcomputers), such as the smallest Apples, Radio Shacks, and Commodores, are not appropriate for most applications discussed here; they are simply not powerful enough and do not possess sufficient memory. For the applications examined in this book, larger computers (those categorized as minicomputers) are assumed to be involved.

In the first chapter, we listed certain alarm bells that signal the need for greater efficiency. Now it's time to roll up your sleeves and examine the specific corners of your practice that may be crying out for electronic help.

Billing and Collecting

To determine and evaluate the initial needs of your business practice, accounts receivables should be studied in depth. What means are used to select, convert, and enter the data into your present system? Are errors easily detected? Are diagnoses and procedures recorded on the financial statements? Is it done by longhand or typewriter? Is it written out or coded? If coded, is it your own code or a universal code? Are all ledger cards up to date with last-minute status information? How are fees generated? Is there any security against a lost charge slip? Are ledger cards frequently misplaced? Are you satisfied with your present system?

Processing all the necessary information manually can be time-consuming. Is the information recorded in a journal and then posted to the patient's ledger? Is it done in one operation or two? Do you have assurances that everything is in balance—charges, payments, and adjustments? How and when are bank deposits prepared?

Does your current system provide an aging analysis? How are delinquent accounts processed to generate income? Is one person responsible for collecting payments on accounts, or is it a combined effort on the parts of several employees?

Computer software can prepare bills; convert CPT (Current Procedural Terminology), ICD (International Classification of Diseases), or other codes for services into statements; produce copies for follow-up billings; produce reminder letters for delinquent accounts; itemize the bills by date, service, and physician; space them out to conform to a cycle billing sequence; analyze accounts receivable by age and by physician; produce a multipurpose claim form (one copy for the patient, one for the insurance company); and fill out insurance forms. This is a minimum start-up package.

Insurance

Insurance billing is probably the most boring job in the office to do by hand, and before long a good medical assistant will decide that there must be more to life than this. Even when using universal claim forms, this is still tedious and time-consuming work. There may be a tendency to start putting it off until tomorrow. And if you rely on insurance company personnel to do the coding on your behalf for diagnoses and procedures performed, you face the likelihood of undetected errors, reduced payment allowances, and claims-processing delays.

Since most patients have some form of medical insurance coverage, it is imperative to have the control of proper coding handled in your office. Relying on an outside source to do this work for you from the brief descriptions recorded on the average claim form can be dangerous and costly.

Are you satisfied with the way your office is handling insurance claim forms? Are your patients happy with the way you are handling their claims? When a claim must be filed over again because of error, your cost of personnel effort increases, there's a delay in generating income, and you've lost some good will in your relationship with that patient.

The patient and the doctor may both be losing money if the insurance companies' payments (allowances for procedures performed) are never questioned. When in doubt, a request for reconsideration can be filed with the insurance company. It's helpful to include substantiating information; for example, if your surgery charge was $1,200 and the allowance was $600, you can request a reconsideration, submitting a copy of your operative report with it. People make mistakes: Your office may have submitted the wrong procedure code; the insurance company may have paid according to the wrong code; the surgery may have been more extensive than usual for the procedure. With a computerized system, checking payments against claims can be easier, and errors or unexpectedly low payments easier to spot.

One doctor who computerized his practice, starting with the insurance billing route, concluded: "If the practice is going to do 40 Medicares and Blue Shields a week, the computer will pay off."

In addition to the potential for payroll savings, computerized insurance claims can reduce the rejection rate by carriers because the data is put in correctly right up front. And the computer can help verify the information on the IRS's 1099-MED forms that come in every year from insurance companies reporting earned income paid to your practice. Without a computer in your office, can you challenge the information on those forms or must you accept it? What recourse do you have? Are there people in your office who can take the time to go back through 12 months' worth of insurance slips to match the totals to the 1099 forms?

Accounting

To the basic billing and collecting software, other computerized accounting functions may be added: accounts payable, general ledger, daysheets, payroll, check-writing, deposit slips, W-2s, and the like. These are less popular than the billing modules, possibly because the payoff is not quite as measurable. A Canadian computer vendor surveyed users and found that only one respondent was using the machine to do payrolls, whereas nearly everyone had computerized insurance claims and accounts receivable. Nevertheless, the computer can not only figure staff pay but calculate doctors' productivity-based pay, no matter how complicated the formula. It will even write the checks.

Many management consultants feel that you can't justify the cost of the accounts-payable/general ledger software (see Chapter 14). Surprisingly, though, your accountant is likely to encourage your purchase. Accountants don't like scut work any better than you do.

Practice Management

REPORTS AND RECORDS. An in-house computer can churn out just about any kind of practice- and financial-management report or summary that you request: practice statistics by income, procedure, physician, or diagnosis; patient profiles by age, location, diagnosis; referral patterns and sources.

In a group practice, for example, some type of record is usually maintained for physicians' productivity (in some case determining salaries or bonuses). Quite often, however, the charges for procedures performed by different physicians are inconsistent. This can be a bad business practice, particularly in view of the fact that patients will sit in the waiting room and discuss or compare charges.

It's also interesting to note that although most practices keep some form of productivity records, not all records reveal the financial adjustments affecting productivity. These adjustments could include, for example, reductions given to a patient after charges have been recorded on his account, or simply the writing off of bad debts.

If your practice has multiple office locations, do you maintain the financial records per location that would be essential to show the cost-effectiveness of each office? Ask these questions:

- Do you need, or would you like to have, additional information per office location?
- If so, what?
- Are financial records kept only at the primary location?
- What system is used to indicate where the business was generated, or who saw the patient?
- Do the physicians rotate between the offices and have certain days to see patients at each location?
- Are charge slips designed to be different for each office location or are they standard for the practice?
- Is there any type of control for the charge slips for the different locations?
- How do you know if a charge slip is lost?
- Are the multiple offices currently causing any problems with your business operation?

OFFICE SUPPLIES AND MAINTENANCE. Efficient operation of any business depends on having the right supplies, in the right quantities, in the right places at the right times. But do you always know what the right supplies are, and what quantities you need? And do you have trouble finding space to store what you've ordered when it comes in?

How good a handle do you have on availability and cost of supplies? Do you have an inventory routine for periodically checking what's available, and a procurement system for requisitioning what you need?

Not all items have equal importance. It would be much more critical to run out of surgical instruments or medicine than out of rubber bands or paper clips. Yet each item must have its place in the system.

A good system lists supplies under various categories, depending on use, such as:

Office supplies
Personalized printed forms
Consumable medical supplies
Drugs and medications
Emergency supplies
Consumable laboratory supplies
Bulk grocery, hardware, and paper items
Patient handouts
Reusable instruments
Reusable medical equipment and supplies
Furniture and accessories.

When you take a close look at the supplies you use, you quickly realize the potential waste of haphazard inventory control—too much is as wasteful as too little, and too little could be hazardous to your patients' (and your practice's) health.

A good inventory should include the level of available supplies, frequency of reordering, and location.

A master inventory list is an invaluable tool. But putting one together is not a one-time process. Is your staff equipped to keep such a list regularly up to date?

As larger-capacity, lower-cost computer memory increasingly becomes available, it may become more and more feasible to use the computer for this purpose. The computer can also be used to prepare requisitions, figure pricing, record orders in the master inventory, and keep the inventory current.

Most important, perhaps, it can rotate orders so that you're able—as often as possible—to take advantage of volume discounts, seasonal price breaks, periodic specials, and the like. And it can maintain a nice balance between having too much capital and space tied up in extra merchandise, and forever worrying that you're about to use your last gauze pad or disposable thermometer. Or that it's the "colds and flu" season, and you're dangerously low on flu vaccine and can't get the detail man on the phone.

Furthermore, the computer can also organize your inventory of reference books and periodicals, and your subscription lists of waiting room reading material. Patients may joke with you about the five-year-old *National Geographics* on your end tables, but they don't always think it's funny.

Appointment Scheduling

Is appointment scheduling a worthwhile use of the computer? Probably not in a solo practice. But in a larger, more complex multispecialty practice, or one with heavy follow-up (such as Ob/Gyn, orthopedic surgery, cardiology), electronic data processing can not only handle appointments efficiently, but can also produce patient reminders and recall lists and even suggest possible evidence for malpractice defense (such as charging a patient with contributory negligence for failing to keep appointments or obtain follow-up care).

But the computer cannot completely replace the appointment book. The appointment book must be available to serve as legal documentation, if needed. It must, of course, be maintained accurately and properly. Erasures are taboo. Everything must be noted in the book, including patients' failure to keep appointments or cancellations of appointments for any reason. And it is the appointment book, not the computer-stored data, that will be saved over the long term.

In order for computer records to be accepted as evidence in court, your security techniques would be examined to prove the data were entered and maintained with absolute accuracy and security. The review method for evaluating the level of security is detailed, since computer records can be altered without leaving any telltale clue. You do have a responsibility to adopt prudent controls; the mere reliance on a computer requires security.

The computer's efficiency in keeping records for daily use is fairly obvious. In addition, it can maximize effective use of doctors' time by allowing staff to see appointments, other obligations, and gaps in the itinerary at a glance. It can also handle external reporting needs, by generating charge slips, records of patients' complaints or symptoms, or other pertinent data.

Clinical Uses

Your automate-or-not decision can't be made without some advance thought of clinical applications. But you have to consider that clinical uses require more storage capacity than a basic financial package—a great deal more, if you contemplate putting histories and physicals or complete medical records into the system. Developing a coding system for physicians' notes may present a problem that should be addressed early on.

It must also be noted that the computer cannot be used to completely replace written records. Written records are needed for legal documentation. But a computerized system can make it possible for the written records to be stored in a "back room," away from the active business office.

PATIENT MEDICAL RECORDS. Providing good health care depends to a great extent on keeping clear, concise, and comprehensive records of diagnoses, treatment, and progress. A clinical record is adequate only if a knowledgeable third party can easily derive from it all pertinent information about a patient's current medical condition and past history. And your practice will run much more smoothly if patient data are neat, easy to refer to, and easily accessible and retrievable.

A physician in a highly specialized practice might keep an adequate clinical record of each patient on one side of a 3 × 5 file card. A primary-care physician, on the other hand, might easily record 20 pages of notes on every patient. Result: bulging files, storage problems, inefficiency.

Efficient filing and retrieval are as crucial to the day-to-day operation of a medical practice as the records themselves. It is as bad to misplace a needed record as to not have one at all.

The problem is that no matter how you or your staff may choose to organize it—alphabetically, numerically, chronologically, active vs. inactive, by treatment—the amount of patient record-keeping proliferates. You end up with an enormous space problem, and the retrieval process becomes increasingly inefficient as the practice grows.

The computer can't eliminate all your file storage space problems, but it can certainly help. It can, for example (depending on the specific system you purchase), permit:

- Organization of records on any basis that makes sense for your practice
- Updating, transferring, or retrieving of records electronically, reducing the need to handle bulky, dog-eared, or torn file folders
- Immediate entry of new-patient material; immediate updating of existing patient records
- Instantaneous retrieval of patient records, by patient's name, code number, etc., or (with some systems) according to diagnosis, medication, or any other feature that may be important to you
- Easy reference to old entries (eliminating the struggle to read the handwriting or shorthand symbols of previous employees)
- Storage of material for as long as desired (depending on your particular system's memory and storage capabilities).

Diagnoses, ICD and/or CPT codes, and information about allergies and drugs can be entered along with billing data at the initial visit—basically a one-minute operation. For systems with full data-base search capabilities, this is essential for minimal searches. If you read an interesting article about right bundle branch block, for example, it's nice to be able to retrieve a list of patients with RBBB to see how your newly acquired knowledge might apply. Or if new information about a drug appears, particularly if it involves newly discovered hazards or a manufacturer recall, it's very helpful to be able to get a quick list of all your patients currently taking that drug.

Storing patient records is only one of the problems in a manual system. In addition to the basic information and treatment chart, a typical patient's file becomes filled with material that is ancillary to or has almost nothing to do with treatment, such as:

Collection reminders
Handouts
Insurance claims
Recall notices and reminders
Referral acknowledgments
Referral requests
Follow-up phone call notations.

Obviously, it would be impractical to use the computer to replace *all* this paperwork. But the computer can replace some of it and make the rest more manageable and less imposing.

MASTER INDEX. In addition to individual patient files, you're probably maintaining a master patient index—the one that tells your medical assistant whether the patient at the desk has seen you before. Since that can make a substantial difference in nature and extent of examination, history required, and fees charged, it's vital that the index be complete and up to date.

In some types of practices, that may be a huge job. Some specialists may tend to see patients irregularly, or at widely spaced intervals. A manually prepared and maintained master index can overwhelm available space if it isn't frequently edited, with aging entries moved to an inactive file or destroyed. And inactive entries that are suddenly reactivated must be reopened, retyped, and refiled if done by hand.

TRANSFERRING RECORDS. A final challenge to record storage occurs when your patient moves, and his records must move with him. Transmitting this kind of information is one of your more ticklish responsibilities. Remember, all information about a patient—whether it's included in medical treatment notes, personal data, or billing records—is privileged and cannot be disclosed without the patient's consent. Before you can send any information along, you must have that consent *in writing*. Even then, there may be times when you can't or don't wish to release information. And once you decide to release anything, your staff has the job of retrieving the data, making a copy for mailing (always keep originals in your office), preparing the forms, typing the appropriate message, and actually mailing it.

And that may not be the end of it. The new doctor may call to question an entry or a treatment—but the substantiating information may have been purged from your active file by that time.

The process is reversed when you're the new doctor requesting information from the previous physician. How often have you been annoyed when the necessary data are late, incomplete, illegible, incompatible with your filing system, or just never forthcoming?

How convenient would it be to have the computer prepare information on departing patients? How efficient would it be to receive easy-to-read printouts from other doctors on all your new patients? How helpful would it be if your computer could talk to other doctors' computers, comparing and exchanging methods of treatment, prescriptions, diagnoses, questions, answers, problems, solutions, and the rest? This may become a reality sooner than you expect.

OTHER CLINICAL APPLICATIONS. Of course, more sophisticated clinical applications of the computer are currently becoming available too (although with a price tag):

• A San Francisco physician offers on-line diagnosis of pulmonary disease through a computerized breath analysis program call PUFF.

• A physician in York, Pa.—with the help of his son, a computer engineer—has developed a sophisticated computerized medical records system. Each afternoon, the computer prints out records for the following day's patients. Each printout lists the patient's last five visits and sets forth the lab work, consultation reports, and other pertinent data associated with them. There's also a medical history, a summary of all past diagnoses and treatments, and a stardard-of-care audit showing the five most recent results of any of 30 different tests (including blood pressure, urinalysis, hemoglobin, etc.).

When a patient arrives for an appointment, a nurse adds worksheets to the record and notes blood pressure, weight, and pulse. After the examination, the doctor writes a treatment plan and, if necessary, passes the record on to one of the pharmacists the group uses. (The record contains a complete history of all the medication the patient has taken, as well as any allergies or other drug reactions.)

After the patient leaves, the worksheet data are entered into the computer automatically updating the patient's file.

Cost: about $100,000. However, the cost of maintaining patients' records has been cut in half.

• A nine-doctor Oklahoma City group, treating 55,000 patients, has a $250,000 system with 25 terminals, four printers, and three remote editing stations. The system provides information needed for swift, accurate diagnosis and treatment.

After each patient visit or hospital discharge, the doctor fills out an encounter slip and dictates his findings. That information, plus lab findings and prescribed medication, is entered in the patient's computerized record. The result: a clear, concise, comprehensive overview of the patient's status that a doctor can scan quickly without having to bother with mounds of extraneous material.

The system aids in the diagnosis and long-term treatment of hypertensive patients by automatically prescribing medication based on data provided by the doctor or a paramedic. A terminal in the hospital emergency room allows the doctors in the group to call up data on clinic patients whenever necessary.

A data base is usually a large and continuously updated file of information on a particular subject that is designed for easy search and retrieval. There are over 200 medically related data bases, with an enormous range of information that may be beneficial to you. For example, AMA NET offers many data bases, as do speciality societies and national health-related centers such as the National Institutes of Health. These data bases are potentially accessible from a computer in your office. For a reasonable cost, a physician with a terminal, a modem, and a telephone can subscribe.

A computer can expand your capacity to make sound decisions. In the not-too-distant future, it's conceivable that you may need to enter a patient's signs and symptoms into a computer so that you do not overlook a possible diagnosis. To do otherwise may simply increase your liability.

With a computer, you also should be able to build your own data base. If, for example, you enter into the system the drugs you prescribe for each patient and a drug is then recalled, you should be able to obtain a list of the patients who are on the medication by pushing a few keys or entering a command into the computer. If, on the other hand, you would like to write an article on a specific diagnosis, you should be able to recall a listing of your patients with that diagnosis for case studies.

Word Processing

Many computer systems include a word processing package as a selling feature. But rarely is such an ancillary package truly adequate for medical office needs. For one thing, the quality of the printing produced by the output device may be sufficient for many typical computer applications, but inappropriate for letters and other word processing uses. If you wish to get involved with word processing in a major way, it's usually best to investigate a separate system.

In any case, the average doctor is often in no hurry to acquire word processing capabilities. That seems to be more the stuff of law firms, banks, and large businesses. But word processing can make life much easier for your staff. Consider:

- How many pieces of communication get typed every week in your office? Just think about all the various and separate kinds of letters to patients; about patients to attorneys, employers, schools, insurers, hospitals, nursing homes, relatives, and other physicians; to other doctors about professional matters; to suppliers, professional associations, community groups, and your various advisers—accountant, attorney, banker, insurance agent, travel agent, and broker.
- How many of these letters are basically identical, except perhaps for a change in the date, addressee, and perhaps a number or phrase somewhere in the letter?
- How many times does your medical assistant have to type the same letters over and over again—repetitiously, tediously—so that Mrs. Jones and Mr. Wilson each get a personal, original letter?
- How often must your assistant tear a nearly finished letter out of the typewriter and start all over because of a typing mistake or a sentence left out of the first paragraph?
- How much of your own time is spent proofreading letters, and how often, then, must your medical assistant type an entire letter over because of a mistake you found?

And think of how much it's costing you to own (or lease), operate, and maintain your copying machine and electric typewriters; and to keep all the related supplies on hand: special paper, toner, ribbons, correcting fluid, opaquing films, etc.

The three basic word processing functions are display, memory, and printing. With these capabilities, you can program certain standard "forms" that you use repeatedly—communications to patients, doctors, insurance companies, etc.—and summon them as needed. Your assistant simply types in the *new* information particular to that letter, and the machine will print an original copy, ready to go.

If she makes a typing mistake she can see it on the screen and can correct it before the letter is actually printed. The machine will make all the adjustments for spacing and line rearranging. Not until the complete letter shows up on the screen as she wants it will it be printed on paper, one time, correctly. Savings: her time and your time, to say nothing of a bundle of wasted supplies.

Is it possible that *you* might need word processing capabilities? Consider how frequently your office must process such standard "boilerplate" documents as:

- Referral letters
- Referral thank-you letters
- Recall notices
- Recall notice follow-ups
- Insurance claim letters
- VA and/or welfare claim letters
- Patient refund letters
- Monthly statements
- Collection letters
- Other letters to patients (appointment changes, authorizations to release medical information, checkup follow-ups, complaint follow-ups, acknowledgments of payment)
- Other letters about patients
- Letters to other physicians about professional matters (congratulations, information replies, information requests, reprint requests, program appearance requirements, speaker invitations)
- Letters to professional associations and journals (membership renewal, requests for information, communications about journal articles submitted)
- Letters to suppliers (catalog requests, invoice errors, order placement, order follow-up, return of defective, unsuitable, or unordered merchandise)
- Letters to your accountant (IRS, bookkeeping, or procedural inquiry)
- Letters to your attorney (incorporation questions, malpractice questions, will update)
- Letters to your banker (questions about bank accounts, IRA, trust, loan, mortgage account).

Does this sound like your practice? Do you still feel that word processing is primarily the concern of the business firm only? Aren't you beginning to see that you're a business, too?

Table 2-2. *How Does Your Current System Compare?*

Look at the features listed below, and compare the performance from your current manual system with what you'd expect to get from a computer. If your current system fails the test, that might be a sign that you have some housekeeping to do before you go computer shopping. By the way, don't assume that the computer will outperform your own system on all these features. And don't take the salesman's word for it either. Check with another physician who owns a computer.

One-minute entry of patient registration into system

Dealing with patient or responsible party as needed

Use of multipurpose billing form

Use of cycle billing

Ability to send out statements on time

Effort at time-of-service payment

Daily preparation of journal

Balancing of daysheets against patient ledgers

Aged accounts receivable reports

Timely collection letters

Daily deposits and posting

Handling of accounts payable on time

Same-day turnaround of insurance forms

Handling of insurance claims and other typing without need for overtime

Automatic audit trail

Account history kept for each patient

Same-day responses to patients' questions

More than one (billing, scheduling, accounting) function handled simultaneously

Personalized notes possible on financial records

Up-to-date correspondence

Quick retrieval of information

Necessity of maintenance contract to keep system in operation

Table 2-2 summarizes some of the areas in which you might wish to compare your current system with what a computer could provide. But remember that a poorly functioning manual system will not be magically improved by acquisition of a computer. Careful planning is necessary to ensure the success of either a manual *or* a computer system.

3. Would It Be Cost-Effective to Computerize?

You've seen ads on television and in newspapers and magazines for computers selling for only a few hundred dollars. You also probably know that you can spend $25,000, $50,000, or more for a computer system for your professional office. Obviously, the $200 or $300 computer won't perform most of the tasks that you'd need for your office (or, for that matter, many of the functions that you'd need in just a home computer). So you'd probably be throwing your money away if you purchased one of these "toy" systems.

But make no mistake: You could also be throwing away your money when you buy an expensive computer system. This doesn't mean just buying the right equipment at the right price (see Chapter 8 for more on this). What it means is that every computer system must be cost-justified. In simple terms, any computer must pay for itself—and more—in actual dollars and cents.

There are three main ways that a computer system can smooth out your practice and thus help put actual dollars in your pocket: (1) by helping to increase productivity, (2) by helping to lower expenses, and (3) by helping to speed up collections.

Increasing Productivity

If a computer system can allow you to see more patients in a day, obviously you can either generate more revenue or spend more time with your family. A computer may enable you to increase your office's productivity by ensuring that you and your assistants are using *your* time as wisely as possible. Instant access to information can cut down the time that you and your assistants must spend with patients. Of course, you won't cut down on your actual diagnostic time, since you still want to continue to give the best possible care. But a computer may allow you to maintain that same level of care while allowing you to see more patients.

Assuming that you opt for increasing revenues, what can you really expect? Let's say that a computer system can increase your daily patient load by 7 or 8 percent through more efficient scheduling and better use of your time. For a physician who is grossing $250,000 a year, that could mean another $18,750—with no increase in usual expenses. If your annual expense for your computer system (the purchase price amortized over a certain number of years plus the actual costs each year) is about $5,000, you'll have netted an extra $13,750 without you, personally, working any harder or having to add any employees to your staff.

Reducing Expenses

Now let's take this same example and examine what a computer might be able to do for your expenses. Let's say that through more efficient purchasing and use of supplies and equipment, you're able to cut your expenses 5 to 6 percent. With a practice that's grossing $250,000, expenses might well run $75,000 to $100,000 or more, depending on your specialty. So if you cut expenses by 5 percent, you could easily save $3,750 to $5,000. And that saving will translate into *net* earnings (before taxes, of course) that can add to your personal income and/or your retirement fund.

The bottom line: By increasing revenues by 7 to 8 percent and cutting expenses by 5 to 6 percent, you might well net an extra $17,500 to $18,750—after paying the annual cost of your computer system. That's quite a sum of money. But speeding up your collections—and increasing the percentage you collect—could add another large chunk to your annual revenues.

Speeding Up Collections

Right now, it's doubtful that you know the average age of your accounts receivable. How old do you think your average bill is? A month? Two months? Four months? And you're probably at least faintly aware that there are some patients' bills that are six or more months in arrears. If none of this worries you, it should. These past-due accounts could be costing you thousands—even tens of thousands—of dollars each year. Maybe you feel that at your income level you should be able to afford that boat you always wanted or that vacation cabin in the mountains—but you never seem to have the ready cash for these things. Well, increasing your collection efficiency could bring you that boat or that cabin.

"But I request payment at time of service," you may be thinking. If so—and *if* most of your patients comply with this policy—the size of your accounts receivable may not be enough to justify the expense of a computer. But if you have difficulty collecting full fees at time of service and you have to send out collection letters, read on.

There are two things to keep in mind when you talk about accounts receivable: (1) the present value of money to be collected at a future date and (2) the probability of collecting a debt as it gets older.

TRUE WORTH OF YOUR ACCOUNTS RECEIVABLE. The present value of money to be collected at a future date is part of the theory of the time value of money. Basically, this theory holds that a dollar collected today will be worth more in the future and that a dollar to be collected in the future is *not* worth a dollar today.

If, for example, someone offered to give you $1,000 today or a year from today, you'd obviously take it today. You know that you can invest that money and earn additional income on it. Even in a bank passbook savings account, you'd earn 5½ percent annually.

But in recent years, investors have been able to earn much more. Money market fund rates, for example, have topped 18 percent annually on occasion. Even with interest rates down and inflation under control, an intelligent investor can earn 10 to 12 percent or more on his money.

So now let's say that you have $10,000 today and you're able to invest it at 12 percent annually—which is about 1 percent per month. It's surprising how fast this sum compounds. At the end of four months, for example, your original $10,000 will have grown to $10,406 (see Table 3-1). After nine months, your $10,000 will have grown to almost $11,000. And at the end of just one year, you'll have $11,268. You'll have this, of course, if you have the $10,000 today to invest.

But remember that your patients can also invest *their* money—instead of paying you. And that's exactly what happens, in effect, when you have accounts receivable. For example, if your accounts receivable total $10,000 and the average age is four months, then you've lost $406 when interest rates are 1 percent per month. That's because you haven't had this money to invest. Even if interest rates shrank to as little as ½ percent per month (about 6 percent annually), you'd still lose over $200 in those four months.

But the best way to look at uncollected revenue is not at what you could earn on it if you had the money in your pocket. What you really have to do is to know the present value of funds to be collected at a later date.

Let's go back to that $10,000 in uncollected receivables that is four months old. Taking a look at the chart in Table 3-2, we can see that when interest rates are 1 percent per month, that uncollected $10,000 is actually worth only $9,610.

Many doctors, of course, have receivables totaling much more than $10,000. Let's say your receivables were actually $50,000 and, once again, they were an average of four months old. Now, based on the 1 percent per month interest rate, that $50,000 is actually worth $48,050. So without even realizing it, you would have been giving your delinquent patients an involuntary discount of almost $2,000.

Table 3-1. *Future Value of $10,000 at Specified Rates of Compound Interest*

Months of compounding	Interest rates (monthly)			
	½%	¾%	1%	1¼%
1	$10,050	$10,075	$10,100	$10,125
2	10,100	10,151	10,201	10,252
3	10,151	10,227	10,303	10,380
4	10,202	10,303	10,406	10,509
5	10,253	10,381	10,510	10,641
6	10,304	10,459	10,615	10,774
7	10,355	10,537	10,721	10,909
8	10,407	10,616	10,829	11,045
9	10,459	10,696	10,937	11,183
10	10,511	10,776	11,046	11,323
11	10,564	10,857	11,157	11,464
12	10,617	10,938	11,268	11,608

Table 3-2. *Present Value of $10,000 to Be Collected at a Future Time at Specified Rates*

Months until collected	Interest rates (monthly)			
	½%	¾%	1%	1¼%
1	$9,950	$9,926	$9,901	$9,877
2	9,901	9,852	9,803	9,755
3	9,851	9,778	9,706	9,634
4	9,802	9,706	9,610	9,515
5	9,754	9,633	9,515	9,398
6	9,705	9,562	9,420	9,282
7	9,657	9,490	9,327	9,167
8	9,609	9,420	9,235	9,054
9	9,561	9,350	9,143	8,942
10	9,513	9,280	9,053	8,832
11	9,466	9,211	8,963	8,723
12	9,419	9,142	8,874	8,615

AGE OF YOUR RECEIVABLES. But there's more. The older an account gets, the less likely you are to collect. If, continuing our example, the average age of your accounts receivable is four months, you may well be able to collect as little as 66 percent of what is owed you.

If that's the case, you can count on getting only $33,000 of the $50,000 due. And that $33,000 will have a present value—at 1 percent a month—of only $31,713. So under these circumstances, you could expect to lose more than $18,000 ($50,000 − $31,713 = $18,287).

HOW A COMPUTER CAN INCREASE REVENUE. A computer system can increase your collection efficiency in several ways. It will give you a current aging analysis of your accounts receivable whenever you want it. It will tell you exactly what this means in lost revenue. And it may be able to generate collection letters as needed, ranging from the first gentle nudge to more demanding requests if the patient continues to fail to pay.

What can this mean to you in dollars in your pocket? Let's keep on with our example. If the computer can help decrease the average age of your accounts receivable to one month, you should be able to collect about 95 percent of what's due you, and you gain the use of that money for three additional months, thereby increasing its present value to you.

Assume you can collect 95 percent of that $50,000; you'll get $47,500. Since this money is discounted for only one month, its present value, at 1 percent per month, is $47,025. So the actual difference computerized collection will make in your pocket will be more than $15,000 ($47,025 − $31,713) over what you could have expected to collect with accounts receivable with an average age of four months.

Of course, the preceding analysis is highly theoretical. You can't count on every dollar to behave so predictably in real life. However, there's enough truth in the underlying theory that almost every big business includes present-value analyses in its major decisions.

In order to decide whether a computer purchase will be cost-justified for you, first analyze your accounts receivable. If your collection ratio is 95 percent and the average age of your accounts receivable is only a few weeks, you may not need a computer system. But this is only one of the areas you should explore in deciding on cost-justification. Here's what to look for and do in putting together an analysis of other significant areas of your practice.

Analyzing Your Costs and Needs

Your analysis of needs and costs will take work and time, and it may ruffle some feathers. You'll have to do some probing in your office. You can't, after all, determine the impact of a computer that can process four insurance claims a minute unless you also know how long your office staff takes to process them by hand.

PROBLEM AREAS TO LOOK FOR. What you'll be looking for are problem areas where the computer can be of help: slow billing, piled-up insurance claims, heavy transcription workload, ineffective patient follow-up and recall, delayed responses to patient inquiries, inadequate management information, confusion about where your referrals are coming from, sluggish cash flow, overworked staff, indecision about adding another physician or opening a new satellite office.

To do your assessment, you need information:

- How many patients you see
- Total number of active patients
- Number of third-party claims, broken down by carrier
- Number of revised claims
- Turnaround for claim payments
- Accounts receivable by account age and physician
- Total daily and monthly posting of charges and payments
- Gross revenues
- Hours or days spent on various office functions.

FIVE-YEAR PROJECTION. You must also estimate your practice expectations for up to five years from the end of your fiscal year. Five-year projections make sense because that's how long the IRS will let you depreciate the hardware you buy. You certainly don't want to commit yourself to such a large capital purchase and annual expense (see Part II) without realistic expectations of being able to handle them easily.

USING A CONSULTANT. A medical practice management consultant might be a good choice to help you develop this information. A good consultant should not have a vested interest in your installing a computer. In fact, an experienced consultant will likely cast a jaundiced eye toward your automating. He's seen too many installations go wrong, and he may even feel that his own services would be more useful to you than any machinery. That's all right. His doubts and cynicism might be a suitable counterweight to your enthusiasm and full-steam-ahead attitude. (And don't be shy about asking him what computer system *his* office employs!)

The best way to find a good medical management consultant in your area is to ask your colleagues for recommendations—especially colleagues of your own specialty and with your type of practice setup. Failing that, you can get names and addresses of reliable consultants in your area by writing to the Society of Professional Business Consultants, 600 South Federal, Chicago, IL 60605, or to the Society of Medical and Dental Management Consultants, 7318 Raytown Road, Raytown, MO 64133.

Guidelines

What guidelines should you use for your evaluation? The obvious answer—"Every practice is different"—is true. But here are a few general yardsticks:

REVENUES. Suggested minimum gross revenues range from as low as $150,000 or $200,000 to $1 million, although some people will tell you, any busy solo practitioner can benefit from a computer. Question them closely. Do they mean a microcomputer or home computer, or are they talking about a more powerful minicomputer system? Again, Part II deals with the specifics of software and hardware capabilities.

As less expensive hardware and better, physician-oriented software are developed and become available, successful installations will be possible at the lower range of size and price for smaller practices. If you feel you're at the low end of the scale, you might rest your decision on your growth plans. If you don't expect your practice to grow much, are happy with present conditions, and don't feel overwhelmed with problems, your decision is easy. Don't computerize your office! Or . . . not yet.

TYPE OF PRACTICE. Naturally, high-volume practices are better candidates for automation than low-volume ones. So family practitioners, general practitioners, internists, pediatricians, Ob/Gyn specialists, and general surgeons with a high component of general practice often generate the volume that makes a computer worth considering. Multispecialty group practices find computers helpful to deal with their complicated productivity and income formulas.

There are exceptions to this guideline. Computers have successfully been placed in practices where the doctor was seeing only about 15 patients a day. Why? Because he was spending upward of $2,500 a month on transcriptions. Word processing is a major attraction in such consultative practices, where long appointments are the norm. A cardiopulmonary group, for example, might have far fewer transactions in relation to gross revenue than a family practice group would, but the cardiopulmonary group's data might be much more time-consuming to process by hand.

LOCATION. Where you practice—and especially your distance from good computer repair service—is another consideration. It's absolutely essential to have someone at the ready who can provide service within hours, not days, if the system breaks down.

For practices that are so remote from major cities that prompt service is difficult, linkage with on-line service bureaus (see Chapter 4) may make more sense than in-house installations.

PAPERWORK. One doctor has decided that at 300 billings per month it's cost-efficient to buy a $15,000 computer system. But those 300 billings might not be a useful benchmark for a practice that works at holding down billings by time-of-service collection. Even physicians whose billings alone can pay for a computerized system should demand a great deal more from the equipment they buy, ranging from searches of medication used by patients to reports of procedure utilization by physician.

Another popular yardstick is that 40 third-party claims a week can make a practice a candidate for an in-house system, although that yardstick wouldn't apply to a practice that makes a strong effort to avoid handling third-party claims. For these reasons, the rate of patient transactions is a better barometer. A good pegboard system, for example, begins to get overloaded at about 300 transactions a day (although some doctors report that volume begins to outstrip the pegboard's ability to handle it at about 150 patients a day in the office plus weekend and hospital visits).

Insurance claim bouncebacks. Insurance claim bouncebacks are another indicator. In practices where the rate reaches 20 or 25 percent, substantial clerical time can be gained by computer software that gets the right information to the carrier every time.

Service-bureau woes. If you now have a service bureau and it's taking four days or more to get a printout in response to a patient query, you might want to consider switching to an in-house computer or an online service bureau. If the system is working properly, you should be able to supply the answer in most cases while the patient is on the phone.

FINANCIAL DATA. We've already discussed how much receivables can cost you. A computer won't eliminate receivables, to be sure, but it's one way your staff can reduce them—especially if statements aren't going out on time, or are going out inaccurately.

NUMBER OF PHYSICIANS. According to some enthusiasts, the minimum number of physicians in a practice that needs a computer is *one* —in other words, any solo doctor is a candidate. A more reasoned approach says four physicians, especially in a primary-care practice. (A group of four surgeons doing advanced procedures, on the other hand, can probably get along nicely on a good manual system.)

PERSONNEL. Consider how hard and how well your staff is working. One of the best times to consider a computer is when you're contemplating hiring another full-time person to handle paperwork—especially insurance forms—because you've scrambled unsuccessfully with part-time help to keep up. Or maybe there's one full-time employee on a posting machine and another doing insurance forms; a computer might eventually enable you to consolidate those two positions into one.

Do your growth plans include bringing in another physician soon? That's a good time to consider a computer, because that extra physician means additional staff effort—and probably personnel. A computer could help you limit your practice to your present staff, or perhaps a part-time addition, and hold down costs.

WORD PROCESSING. In evaluating your need for word processing, focus on professional time as well as staff time. Doctors, after all, must compose, edit, and review the letters, reports, and articles that go out on their letterheads. Remember, too, that the medical assistant who does typing isn't *always* typing. She might also be filing, answering the phone, scheduling your appointments, or doing a variety of nontyping chores. Word-processor capability can free much of an assistant's time for these other chores.

General Conclusions

Your needs analysis should lead you to some general conclusions. For example:

- You have a good manual system, but it can't keep up with the volume of your practice
- Your present system is handling your current volume right now, but you have an aggressive growth plan for your practice
- Your present system is unsound, and you have to do something to get things squared away.

In any of these circumstances, you should definitely look into a computerized system (see Table 3-3). The odds are very good that

Table 3-3. Cost Analysis Worksheet

Item	Your figures	Sample figures
Costs		
Hardware		$ 10,000
Software		6,000
Total		16,000
Less tax saving from five-year depreciation and investment credit		(9,280)
Net after-tax cost		6,720
Software modifications		0
Modem and other attachments		200
Consultant		4,000
Cost of continuing manual system (labor × months)		2,400
Insurance increase		500
Site preparation		500
(continued)		
Projected practice growth rate	____%	10%
Projected payroll over five years at current percentage of gross		427,357
Projected payroll over five years at target percentage of gross		366,306
Payroll savings over five years		61,051
Average accounts receivable 60 days or older		20,000
Five-year earnings on additional collections (invested @ ___%)		7,623 (12%)
Total savings over five years (payroll + accounts receivable)		**68,674**

Total	**14,320**
Monthly cost over five years (÷ 60)	239
Service or maintenance contract	200
Additional personnel	1,200
Total monthly cost of system	**1,639**

Projected savings

Current payroll and percentage of gross revenues	(%)	$ 70,000 (14%)
Target percentage of gross revenues	%	12%

Projected monthly savings (÷ 60)	1,145
Plus savings in accounting and consulting fees	200
Net projected monthly savings	1,345
Monthly projected cost	1,639
Less cost of additional person	1,200
Net projected cost	439
Net monthly savings (or added expense)	**906**

such a move will be very cost-effective. You'll have to realize, though, that a computer can't organize a disorganized practice. Before a computer can start making it more effective, you'll have to get it organized for maximum efficiency. That's a job best entrusted to an experienced practice management consultant.

Then there's one other conclusion that you can reach: Your present system works just fine and can handle any extra volume that you think you might generate. In that case, you may not need a computer. So don't be in any rush to run right out and get one.

4. Service Bureaus: A Wise Alternative?

The advantages of a computer should be obvious to you by now. The disadvantages may be obvious as well—the $20,000 on up (and maybe beyond $100,000) that you'll have to spend on the hardware and software.

To minimize the initial costs, especially when the practice is just groping its way into EDP (electronic data processing), many consultants recommend using outside service bureaus.

A service bureau is basically an outside commercial firm with a full complement of equipment and more computer capacity than it's currently using. It will lend this capacity to you—not just the equipment, but any applicable programs it has available plus any systems planning it has in-house—for a charge. By making all this capability available, it frees you of a lot of the costs and headaches of computerization. It may also deprive you of some of the advantages of in-house EDP as well.

What Service Bureaus Do

THE BASIC MENU. Some service bureaus specialize in working with medical practices, but most will offer only a basic menu of the things you need: billing and accounting services. You provide them with your data, and they'll return to you up-to-date financial statements, completed insurance forms, employee payroll materials, checks to suppliers and outside parties, complete transaction and account records, and the like. Some also provide a broad range of additional services, including storage of medical records, direct access to third-party payers, preparation of practice profiles, inventory control, appointment scheduling, patient-recall systems, and word processing.

ADVANTAGES. Not only do service bureaus offer lower initial costs, EDP expertise, and less space requirements, but any downtime is the service bureau's problem, not yours.

In a world of rapidly changing computer technology, use of a service bureau could prevent your acquiring an in-house system soon to become obsolete. And it can also keep you up to date with the latest software. Programming is one of the major problems, and also one of the major costs, of a new, private, start-up computer installation.

DISADVANTAGES. However, service bureaus also come with certain disadvantages:

- The time they require to process and verify your information may not fit your needs.
- You lack flexibility in choosing software applications for your practice; many service bureaus require doctors to adapt their systems to the bureaus' capabilities.
- You have practically no control over computer usage.
- You risk sacrificing confidentiality by sending your records outside your office.
- In most cases, you lack instant access to the mainframe equipment.
- You don't get the tax credits and depreciation you would if you bought your own system.
- You still need trained personnel in your office who are at least familiar with computer jargon and operations. And if what you are buying is on-line time sharing on the bureau's equipment (see below), your personnel must be trained to actually operate the system.
- You're usually locked into a specified schedule of processing.
- Computer use is usually limited.
- You always run the risk that the service bureau may eventually go out of business.

And then there's the *ransom factor*. If a service bureau does go out of business, or learns that you don't plan to renew your contract, it may make it very difficult for you to retrieve your records from its computer storage.

COSTS. Costs must be justified whatever you do. In the case of a service bureau, an initial cost is charged for each account entered into the system, and that cost depends on whether your employee enters the data or it's done by the service bureau's personnel. In addition, there are charges per transaction, per insurance form, per statement, per line of report, per report, per error correction, and for mailing, equipment, telephone lines, access time, and storage—plus some minimum monthly charge.

How Service Bureaus Work

Service bureaus work in three basic ways:

1. ON-LINE TIME SHARING. Through your own terminal (and usually a printer), you're tied directly to the service bureau's mainframe, which gives you, in effect, in-house computerization. But you share access with other users, which means you may not have all the access you require whenever you require it. (It's something like having a telephone party line.) However, most large service bureaus can provide what amounts to unlimited access, with very few restrictions.

2. ON-LINE SERVICING. You have your own terminal, maybe with a printer, both of which allow you to communicate directly with the service bureau's computer. But all you can do is send, and in some cases receive, information. You supply the service bureau with the raw data, and it provides the reports, statements, invoices, paychecks, claim forms, and the rest. No expertise or major equipment is required of you, but neither do you have any flexibility. You're limited by the service bureau's programming capabilities, and also by the service bureau's speed in turning your work around.

3. OFF-LINE BATCH PROCESSING. This is the simplest and least expensive way to use a service bureau. Your staff fills out transaction forms, sends them to the service bureau (usually in daily batches, either by mail or messenger), and you receive the work back, typically in 48 hours, again by mail or messenger. The advantages are clear: no capital outlay, a minimum of staff training, no space requirements, and all data entry done by off-premises professionals who are likely to be more highly trained than the personnel in a doctor's office. And the costs are reasonable—generally about $1.00 per active account per month, without the additional few hundred (or even thousand) dollars per month in equipment leasing and maintenance required in the first two arrangements.

Some experts recommend off-line batch processing for low-volume users requiring 1,500 or fewer statements a month. Others feel it's the best system regardless of practice size (perhaps other than buying an in-house system). But there are some negatives. A batch system requires that data be prepared twice, once in your office format and once for the computer. Furthermore, you have no immediate way of answering a patient's question about his bill while the transaction forms are away being processed.

Other Variations Service Bureaus Offer

CONTRACT A/R MANAGEMENT. Contract accounts-receivable (A/R) management takes almost all of the billing paperwork out of the medical office, and offers follow-up on outstanding accounts, office staff training, management advice, and even the handling of patient inquiries. Charges usually range from 6 to 16 percent of collections, depending on volume.

DISTRIBUTED DATA PROCESSING. In this variation, daily tasks such as patient-account processing, insurance invoicing, and patient scheduling are handled through an in-house minicomputer, while statement printing and other functions are performed by the service bureau's mainframe computer.

COMMUNICATION COSTS. All these variations except off-line batch processing may involve substantial communication costs—unless the service bureau or host computer is within range of a local telephone call. (For computer-access purposes, a phone call within the area of your local telephone directory—let alone your area code—may not be considered "local." Check with the service bureau *and* your telephone company to make sure telephone-access charges won't be levied—or, if they will, you may want to shop around for a service bureau that allows you cheaper telephone access.) That's a strong argument for favoring a service bureau with an office close to yours, but it isn't the only one. A nearby office is accessible not only for routine procedural matters but also when something goes wrong. If your bills haven't gone out, for example, or your receivables report is overdue, you'll prefer dealing with someone around the corner to shouting into a long-distance telephone connection.

Standard Billing Functions
Handled by All Systems

With all billing systems, certain standard functions must be performed:

* Initiating and updating patients' accounts
* Storing historical information
* Posting transactions
* Reconciling financial data
* Billing patients
* Processing insurance claims
* Reporting financial information.

The service bureau must be able to perform these functions in a timely manner, so it must have a special program to handle the needs of a medical office.

COMPLETING FORMS AND PROCESSING DATA. To initiate or update patient-account records with batch processing requires your staff to complete the forms provided by the service bureau and return them for entry into the bureau's computers. There's a time lag between completing the forms and processing the data. If you're on line, your staff enters the data directly via the computer terminal in your office. But you may not be able to receive an audit trail—hard copy of transactions entered into the computer—when the work is completed. And without this paper record, it may be very difficult to detect errors.

INFORMATION STORAGE, ACCESS, AND UPDATING. Historical information is visit-by-visit data kept on patients' ledger cards; computer systems store this information electronically. While computer storage is expensive, you've probably decided at this point that you must have it—and the bigger your practice, the greater your need. You must have access to patients' financial records for at least the previous year. Both batch and on-line service bureaus should provide detailed listings of your patients' accounts on a periodic basis.

ENCOUNTER FORMS. Encounter forms are used for posting transactions. It's usually best to have separate encounter forms for charges, payments, and adjustments. With batch processing, the forms are completed and forwarded to the service bureau. On-line, your staff makes the entries directly.

TOTALS. Totals accompany the entry of encounter forms, and the service bureau compares the submitted totals with its own calculations. A batch summary listing is provided by the service bureau and returned to you for corrections, if necessary. This functions as your audit trail of posted transactions. If you subscribe to an on-line service, the reconciliation process is performed at the terminal. It may require the operator to enter the total before the computer total is displayed, or the operator may simply be asked whether all entries are correct.

BILL PREPARATION. Patients' bills are usually prepared on high-speed printers (both for batch processing and for most on-line servicing) and then mailed either directly to the patients or back to the medical office for mailing. Some on-line service bureaus produce patient statements on a printer located in the medical office.

Universal Insurance Claim Form

Most automated systems generate the universal claim form. Some also meet the special requirements of major third-party payers. Some systems may even submit claims directly to the insurance carriers on magnetic media or via telephone lines. It's essential that you know how any prospective service bureau works in the generation and submission of insurance claims.

Detailed Reports

Computerized service bureaus can produce many detailed reports (see Chapter 19), which can be customized to meet specific requirements. You do, however, pay for the reports on a unit basis. So you ought to know which ones you need and are worth paying for, and which ones you can live without. You should also know how the service bureau's computer releases these reports. If they're done on microfiche, you'll need to buy or lease a microfiche reader.

Control Over Your Service Bureau

One of the oft-repeated caveats about using a service bureau is loss of control. To some physicians, that means not having the ability to control the input into and output from the computer system. Your hesitancy regarding service bureaus, however, should extend far beyond that vague consideration.

When you use a service bureau, after all, confidential medical information is transmitted from your office without signed authorization for release of the information to an outside firm. If it's done by mail, it could be lost. You must decide whether or not you have the confidence in the service bureau to justify entrusting it with such confidential information. You wouldn't hire just anyone to work in your office, and you must exercise the same judgment when selecting an outside service bureau.

General Criteria to Look For

BASIC CONSIDERATIONS. What other criteria should you use in selecting a service bureau? You probably should shun one that hasn't been in business at least three years. Also look for one that specializes in medical and dental practices.

Stay away from one that's affiliated with a bank or computer manufacturer. If the parent company suddenly needs computer capacity, the bureau's clients will suffer. And, of course, try to find a bureau with offices close to your own, as mentioned above.

You must also find out how charges are computed. There could be a fee for conversion of your present system. Most bureaus charge a fee for each active account, and they may also charge a fee for each insurance form processed, each statement rendered, and each report issued. There will probably be a charge for correcting errors and reporting the corrections. Then you may be charged a basic charge, plus a fee for supplies, postage, and any telecommunications.

REMAINING HOMEWORK. Once you find a service bureau that seems to be worth a second look, do some homework before making any commitments:

- Ask for references, and check out the bureau's reputation with two or three physician-clients—preferably doctors with practices similar to yours.
- Ask your bank or other credit source to verify the firm's financial stability.
- Visit the main office. Make sure there's a fireproof vault or cabinet for storage of your records.
- Find out whether the bureau carries insurance to protect you against loss by fire or theft.
- Determine what steps will be taken to guarantee the confidentiality of your records.
- Examine the forms your staff will have to use, and have your staff look at them too, to see that they're clear and simple.
- Satisfy yourself that the firm has adequate computer backup in case its equipment breaks down.
- Ask about turnaround time for processing, and find out who pays postage on outgoing bills.

Above all, don't let your guard down simply because you decide to use a service bureau rather than buy a computer. Contracting for services that you don't need, or failing to make use of available services that you do need, can turn service-bureau computerization into a curse rather than a blessing for your practice.

5. Don't Forget
the Human Factors

Cost is by no means the only consideration in computerizing. At least as important is the inevitable confusion and trauma that will occur among your office personnel who must face their first involvement with electronic data processing.

Change is always traumatic, and the success or failure of your installation will rest on how well you prepare your personnel to accept and adapt to the system.

WHY COMPUTERS ARE UNPOPULAR. Five common reasons for computer system failures are often cited:

1. Lack of support from the boss
2. Failure to appoint a good computer administrator with leadership abilities
3. Failure to keep the staff fully informed as to how the change will affect each one of them
4. Failure to provide adequate training
5. Failure to manage the system.

If your employees don't want a computer, they'll find a way to make sure it doesn't work. So you'll have to sell your staff on the idea before the first piece of hardware arrives. The more your people understand how the system will help them, the more their resistance will diminish. And the more they know that they'll have adequate time to be trained on the machinery, to learn about its capabilities, and to know what's coming in general, the more their fears will be allayed.

Fear of change. Just what fears are we talking about? First of all, fear of change. It affects everyone, at one time or another. The unknown looms, causing hesitation and clinging to the status quo. To overcome it, there must be a leader who can persuade the hesitant that they can cope successfully with whatever comes.

Fear of failure. Fear of failure will also cause personnel to resist change. So if a computer is wheeled into your office without the proper steps having been taken, it will almost surely be shot down by your employees and doomed to fail! Your people will no longer feel secure in their positions, but will fear loss of their job security, professional growth, and salary increases—and they'll exert every effort to prove the computer won't work.

Your Leadership Role

SELLING YOUR ASSOCIATES. Surprisingly, if you're in group practice, the first signs of resistance may come not from your staff but from some of your associates. They are the first to be involved, so if you're leading the way, you must be not only a super-salesman but also a leader who is willing to uphold the objectives of progress and counteract the resistance.

Your associates will resist the computer primarily because it's a costly venture and because they've heard so many stories about computer systems that failed. Don't underestimate their opposition. Their attitude can create havoc. And disagreement among physicians has a way of revealing itself throughout the office. Any sign of a negative attitude among the doctors will permeate the staff—almost a sure guarantee that the system won't work.

If you computerized your office over 5 years ago, you may still meet resistance from your associates to upgrade the system or get a new system to accommodate the major changes that have occurred more recently. The attitude may be, "If it isn't broke, don't fix it." But the ground you're losing by keeping your old system in operation may be costly in many ways.

The changes can cause you to take your current system to paper before implementing a new system, or you may find there's so much manual intervention with your current system that you have lost sight of your original objectives for getting a computer in the first place.

STIMULATING STAFF CONFIDENCE. Physicians must display confidence in their decision—and in their staff—to influence positive action and performance from their employees. Keep your doubts and infighting behind closed doors. Present a united front.

While your colleagues are concerned with costs, and with the chance of failure, your office personnel will resist because they're the ones most directly affected by the change—to an extent they probably don't even anticipate—and because they feel responsible for successful implementation and future results. But the resistance on both fronts will be less if proper assurance is given that careful shopping will keep costs and mistakes down, and that staff personnel will continue to be actively involved during the decision-making, selection, and change-over periods.

If you're the spearhead of the effort to change, you'll have to maintain your involvement and leadership throughout the process. Too many doctors feel their responsibility ends at the time the financial decisions are made. But you must remain actively involved at least until your management people have overcome their fears and are ready to lead the rest of the staff.

Now, more than ever, your leadership and insights are needed. You must understand your colleagues, assistants, and their personal goals, and find a way to intertwine those goals with the fulfillment of your objectives.

Convince them that a change can be exciting and challenging, rather than dreaded and feared, if it's handled properly.

Group Training Sessions

With the proper guidance, group training sessions can be almost thera-peutic. They provide a "we're-all-in-this-together" feeling, and a posi-tive stimulus to mutual help. It's the old-fashioned spirit of teamwork, of everyone working together toward the same objectives.

STIMULATING PERSONAL CONFIDENCE. Employees should be given the opportunity to express their personal feelings and ideas. And you should take the opportunity not only to evaluate those feelings and look for new ideas that could be helpful to the computer installation, but also to radiate enthusiasm. But don't overlook negative factors; they should be examined, as it may be necessary to incorporate addi-tional changes into your plans to help guarantee a smooth transition. In short, treat the staff as the most important consultants in your prac-tice. A ploy? Not necessarily. Your future, or at least the future of your computer, depends on your staff's acting in your best interests.

Feel as if the Battle Hymn of the Republic ought to be playing softly in the background? Perhaps. But countless physicians, and other busi-nessmen as well, have sat in the rubble of their computer disasters wondering what went wrong. And what went wrong, as often as not, was failure to consider the human element. In more medical offices than you can imagine, computers are gathering dust. Why? Because the actual users—the office assistants—were never consulted, never given an opportunity for any input. They were simply handed a fait accompli and expected to make the damn thing work. But if the operator doesn't believe the system will work, it won't, no matter how good it is or how carefully it was selected.

GETTING STAFF INPUT. Naturally, *all* personnel can't be involved in the selection of a computer, but they can be kept informed—and at least the key people should be given an opportunity to try some of the available systems and to voice their opinions. A couple of things will then happen: Since these are the people who best understand office procedure, you'll likely end up with the system that will work best for you. Plus, you've begun to convince the users that the change will be beneficial for all concerned. They'll begin to realize that the change can actually heighten their positions, skills, and salary potentials, and the fears regarding job security will begin to decrease.

DISCUSSION AND ORIENTATION SESSIONS. To give your position maximum credibility, point out all the benefits and be as specific as possible. Talk with each medical assistant in private, addressing yourself to her own position. Emphasize that there are few occupations or professions requiring as many different skills as medical assistants are required to perform, and now you're adding electronic data processing to the list. Let your office team know that you realize the transition will be extremely difficult at times, and you expect them to have problems and even, at times, to fail. Alleviate fears before they are expressed.

But let the staff know that there will be orientation sessions and discussions, training time will be provided for those directly involved in the operation, and everyone will be an integral part of the overall success. Your willingness to help your employees increase their skills, as well as acquire new ones, can be presented as a challenging opportunity. Psychologists say that learning new skills is a strong motivator for employees. Take advantage of this excellent chance to benefit both your employees and the practice, and present the computer learning challenge positively.

Your Computer Administrator

You can't be expected to carry on the computer-leadership role forever. You have patients to minister to; besides, you should become less and less involved in the actual running of the computer as time goes on. However, some *one* person must be in charge of the computer system; identify or acquire a computer administrator early. This will not necessarily be a separate, full-time person with no additional duties. But one person *must* be the leader.

QUALIFICATIONS. The selection process may not be easy. This person must be someone who:

1. Is a leader
2. Can sell your ideas and act in your behalf

3. Understands the personal goals of each individual in the office and can assist in attaining them
4. Completely understands the current manual system
5. Understands what can be accomplished with the prospective computer system
6. Has some business background as well as management skills
7. Has judgment abilities you're comfortable with (particularly since there will be times when a decision must be made on the spot)
8. Is competent and confident, not afraid of change or the problems that might arise as the direct result of change
9. Is willing to learn everything possible about your office computer
10. Is willing and able to help teach others.

This competent leader should radiate an attitude of confidence while making the people who are performing the tasks feel needed, important, and appreciated. Having the appropriate leadership qualities will help assure that objectives are achieved, usually with the least cost, effort, or resistance from those involved.

RESPONSIBILITIES. Your computer administrator must also accept responsibility for others, since achieving the overall objectives for the computer system is the obligation of the position. That obligation is ongoing; efficiency must be maintained at all times. All future changes for the medical office may affect the computer system, as will the future growth of the practice, and any changing technology.

There's a premium, too, on willingness to work long hours, particularly in the early stages and whenever problems develop. Certainly, not just anyone can be placed in this position if you expect good results from your investment.

SOURCES. Where do you find this paragon? It may not be easy. Excellent technical skills or a high rating for on-the-job performance does not necessarily qualify someone for an administrative position. In fact, doing a job well is an entirely different thing from teaching someone else how to do it well; and doing and teaching a job well don't necessarily qualify someone to make sure subordinates measure up to the same standards.

In-house personnel. There are advantages, to be sure, with selecting someone from your present office staff—familiarity with the system and with the other personnel and patients, and a sense of relief when the other employees feel things won't be changing too drastically.

Outside sources. But you might have to go outside to get your computer administrator. As more and more medical practices computerize, there is a growing pool of technically proficient administrators who specialize in medical systems, who have gone through one or more conversions and know the special problems that can and do occur. A computer administrator must be able to communicate with the computer company's personnel—salesmen, programmers, systems analysts, field engineers—so must have the kind of technical knowledge and experienced know-how that you're not likely to find on your staff.

CMA. A certified medical assistant (CMA) with an accounting and administrative background could fill the bill for you. Certification is a voluntary program offered by the American Association of Medical Assistants and administered through the National Board of Medical Examiners. An examination is given covering medical terminology, anatomy, and physiology; human relations, psychology, and economics; medical law and ethics; administrative and clinical procedures.

Simply taking the test indicates confidence and ambition on the part of your applicant. Passing it indicates more-than-minimum competence in those areas.

Degree programs. In addition, you can look for graduates of a two-year associate-degree program in medical assisting; and for those who've had experience in medical-office management, accounting, or business administration—especially in an office that has recently undergone automation.

All things considered. If you still feel most comfortable selecting someone from your current staff, remember that work experience in data processing—while helpful—is not mandatory. An aggressive individual who is knowledgeable about the practice can always learn the necessary computer technology by attending seminars, talking with vendors, reading, or meeting with office personnel from other computerized medical practices.

TRAINING YOUR COMPUTER ADMINISTRATOR. To further her education, she can enroll in post-secondary courses in data processing offered at most local colleges, adult education facilities, and the like.

Many doctors who have undergone the experience feel that it's much easier to teach data processing and data-processing management to a competent medical-office employee than it is to teach the operations of a medical office—procedures, terminology, law, ethics, etc.—to someone with a college degree in business and/or experience in data processing.

Using a Consultant

Whatever your computer administrator's background, involve her from the very beginning, when you first begin shopping for systems. That way, she can begin to learn from the demonstrations given to you. An outside management consultant who specializes in computer installations can help bridge the gap as both you and your administrator are learning the ropes. If you don't really know what you're looking for and what questions to ask, all systems will look attractive. A consultant (see Chapter 3) should be able to assist you in selecting a system, by pointing out the differences in various programs, noting benefits *and* disadvantages, and helping you find the one that best suits your needs and budget.

Of course, consultants charge handsomely for their services, so be sure you're getting your money's worth. Check references, and ask especially for the names of medical practices that have undergone successful computer conversion with the consultant's help. Try to find a consultant who will not abandon you once the system has been selected, but will assist you through the entire installation and implementation period. And avoid a consultant who is pushing a particular manufacturer or supplier, or one who has a connection with a manufacturer or supplier, no matter how he tries to minimize it.

Your Continuing Involvement

Does your involvement and leadership end once the computer administrator has taken over? Hardly. A change like this, which affects the entire office, depends continually for its success on the doctor's involvement. You must be leader and listener, but above all you must be supporter of the change.

To be productive, of course, physicians must practice medicine and delegate other duties to the staff. But that doesn't mean that they should completely remove themselves from office management.

COORDINATING STAFF EFFORTS. You've picked the computer. You can't now simply drop it like a hot potato into the laps of others, even with the presence of a skilled computer administrator. Knowing the advantages that you expect from your computer system should be enough to keep you actively involved, supporting the staff and the system you selected. Your support will be especially vital when problems are encountered—and they will be—and when the system will not do what you thought it would, or in the way you expected.

Problems will occur, and options will have to be discussed. Selecting the best way to handle these situations is usually the job of the computer administrator. Your responsibility is to resist bad-mouthing the system and heading off similar efforts by your colleagues and employees. An employee who has soured on the system—or at least makes noises as if he has—will soon be identified as a weak link. Employees will seek him out to complain about all minor problems, blowing them into major ones. This leads only to further sourness and complaining. Before long, the computer system is doomed to failure. And then it sits, gathering dust like so many of its brethren.

MAINTAINING MORALE. But keep the problems at the management level—or, better yet, help the computer administrator head them off— and staffers will most likely keep working along trying to do their jobs and accomplish their goals.

A computer system can be the best investment you'll ever make in terms of providing good patient care and increasing office efficiency. But it's no panacea.

No computer system is completely satisfactory for everyone, nor will it fulfill every dream. At times, gloom and frustration will predominate. Demands will be unrealistic, and staff dissatisfaction will boil over. Face reality and accept the facts of what a computer can and cannot do for you. Air frustrations and discuss problems with your computer administrator; even call in the manufacturer's or vendor's service representative. Find workable solutions rather than letting gripes fester.

Even when everything appears to be going relatively well, significant problems may lurk offstage. Try to be prepared for them. A positive influence can create positive action. Once you've made a commitment to automation, don't abandon it for a moment or your chances of successful implementation will decrease rapidly.

SUMMARY OF HUMAN ELEMENTS. It's most important to remember all the human elements involved in making the change to a computer system rewarding:

1. Keep your personnel informed and involved, and they'll be interested in working toward the success of their future and yours.
2. Evaluate their feelings collectively and individually; that will provide you with essential information to help guarantee a smooth transition.
3. Understand that your employees will be affected by the computer system and, in return, they will affect the system and its overall success.
4. Stay actively involved, as counselor, cheerleader, teacher, father figure, and consoler.
5. Recognize that human elements play an important part in implementing change; this will help pave the way for positive action and greater achievements.

Above all, remember that accomplishments are a wonderful incentive for continuing to move ahead. The office team should now be ready for appropriate training to make it all happen successfully—for their welfare, for the welfare of the practice, and for yours.

As the actual day approaches for delivery of your computer system, the pace of your staff's involvement accelerates. This phase is further discussed in Chapter 14.

II. How to Get the Right Computer System for You

6. Keeping Pace with Third-Party Payers

If third-party payers aren't drastically affecting your business operations, they soon will be. According to *A Reader's Digest Report to Consumers: Should You Join an HMO?*, August 1987, "Health maintenance organizations are rapidly overtaking insurance plans as America's most popular healthcare system." Can insurance plans overtake a health-care system? Probably not! But the plans do affect the way you practice and critically impact on your business operations. In other words, if you don't practice by the rules, you don't get paid! (See the Preface.)

The impact of prepaid health care on the fee-for-service practice is significant and has many effects. But let's examine how some of the changes are affecting the business side of the practice. Primary care physicians have been affected by capitation, whereas the specialists have been affected by discounted fee-for-service. Consequently, the major impact has been on bookkeeping, claim processing, and billing procedures. The accounting system used in the past may not be the information system needed today. Many practices, however, have been so busy coping with the changes that they haven't had the time to evaluate all the effects.

Prepaid medicine has also caused health-care indemnity plans to change. In an effort to lower the cost of insurance premiums, the patient's cost-share (deductible and co-payments) has increased significantly. The patient must exercise utilization control in the same way that the practice must exercise utilization control under capitated medicine. The indemnity plans offer the subscriber freedom of choice for selecting their physicians, whereas HMOs contract with employer groups, hospitals, physicians, pharmacies, etc. If you retain a standard fee-for-service practice, as well as the right to contract with as many prepaid health-care plans as you desire, you'd better be prepared to manage a system that produces the maximum amount of cash in the shortest possible time at reduced associated costs.

What type of insurance benefits does the patient have? You need to know, and it needs to be recorded. For example, the deductible may be $100 and the co-payment $10. This means the patient is responsible for paying the first $100 of covered medical expenses and then $10 for each office visit. The patient also may have a co-payment for special procedures, such as injections, lab work, x-ray, etc. Does your system allow you quick access to this type of information? Will a computer system allow entry of the data? Remember—a computer should enhance your collection procedures.

It's almost mandatory to file an insurance claim for every procedure performed. Everyone knows that a computer excels in generating insurance claims. In return, most insurance companies provide an explanation of benefits (EOB)—and hopefully a check—in response to the claim. For example, the EOB shows charge(s) submitted, amount allowed, deductible amount, co-payment, and the payment. Does your manual system or computerized system allow for the entry of this information?

If it's necessary to obtain precertification of hospital admissions or approval of your treatment plan, does your system allow for entry of authorization numbers? Under capitated medicine, the primary care physician must provide the specialist with an authorization number when requesting an evaluation for the patient. The number is essential for billing; in fact, the bill must be presented on the claim form designated by the health-care plan and should include statistical and medical data as well as patient data and any identifying information required by the plan. It must also be submitted within a specified number of days from the date of treatment.

Are you beginning to realize that the practice's profit is determined by the effectiveness and efficiency of the physicians and their staffs? Do you see how important it is to select a computer system that can handle your present and future needs, as far as application software? Do you realize the need for selecting a reliable vendor who will provide program enhancements for keeping the practice up to date and/or current with the times?

Many programs written in the past simply can't handle the billing procedures required today. Too much change has occurred. An obsolete program will hinder the efficiency of the practice. The more outdated the program becomes, the more difficult it may be to change systems. You may not be able to transfer the data electronically from one system to another but instead will have to dump the information to paper and then key it into the new system. Since change will probably be essential, you'll need to prepare for it.

DRGs have affected hospital billing procedures and corresponding payment. What if, all of a sudden, you had to incorporate DRG billing? This possibility is under study.

The AMA universal claim form is now accepted by about 90 to 95 percent of insurance carriers. What if a major carrier announces a totally new claim form for submitting information that calls for more detailed information than the data required on the universal claim form? It just recently occurred in Virginia, with traumatic effects.

Blue Cross-Blue Shield of Virginia now requires all their providers to submit claims on a new form with extensive changes, requesting far more information than other insurance companies need. The forms are processed by an optical scanner, and, according to the Blues, this new technology is more efficient, etc.

The change has created chaos—and rightly so. The claim form for billing Blue Cross-Blue Shield plans throughout the country has never been standardized. Consequently, the sweeping changes Blue Cross-Blue Shield of Virginia has made for filing their claims is a local problem. *It should demonstrate, however, that this situation can happen anywhere at any time!*

In response to the provider's concern, Blue Cross/Blue Shield of Virginia has more recently announced that they will accept the universal claim form, but they also have warned the providers that claims submitted on this form may reject because of insufficient information. Thus, you might ask, "Is this a viable solution?" It certainly doesn't appear to be. Rejected claims cause cash flow to decrease and expenses to increase.

Medical practices that have previously computerized their business operations may be in a state of turmoil. Some computer systems cannot accommodate the changes. Reliable computer vendors are trying to stay abreast of national or regional issues that affect the business operations of a medical practice—and understandably so. But in the Commonwealth of Virginia, a major insurance carrier has made drastic changes for submitting claims, and the computer vendors are trying desperately to enhance their program to accommodate them; however, it may not be a win-win situation. Certainly the physicians will have increased costs associated with all the changes.

The providers who are on a manual system are having their problems, too. The optical scanner will only read a typewritten or computer-generated form. The form must line up perfectly. Any extraneous characters or less-than-perfect alignment can cause the claim to reject. The solo physician has just about reached a point in time to decide whether or not he/she can continue to cost-justify a manual system.

To complete the new form, additional information must be obtained and recorded. For example, if a patient is seen relative to an accident, not only must the date of the accident be recorded but also the time the accident occurred and the time the physician rendered treatment. This is the case for medical emergency, accident, or follow-up accident care.

Coding information on the new form has also changed. For instance, on the AMA universal claim form, the subscriber is identified by the patient's relationship to subscriber code of 01. The new claim form for the Blues *requires* a 2-alpha character code; for example, EE indicates the subscriber. Many computer systems—or the application software—may not be able to handle the change. Can the patient's relationship to subscriber file be expanded? If so, can the computer transfer the patient relationship to subscriber code 10, for example, to print EE? If so, you now have a system that can accommodate the change, but you also have a system that increases the chance of human error for data entry. When entering patient data for patient relationship to subscriber code, do you enter 01 or 10 to identify that the patient is the subscriber? You now have two sets of does for identifying the needed information. When a patient changes insurance carriers, this information must be checked for accuracy of the two coding systems.

The new form requires the 3-digit ICD-9 diagnosis codes and will accept up to 5 characters. But you cannot key or type the decimal. The ICD-9 uses the decimal to better define the diagnoses for all insurance carriers. If you're currently computerized and use the ICD-9 diagnosis codes, the diagnosis file for your practice should have been built accurately—using the decimal, if needed. If the decimal prints on the new claim form for Blue Cross-Blue Shield of Virginia, the claim apparently will reject. The instructions are *not* to use the decimal. Does this make good sense? Do you understand how a computer system that was working effectively yesterday cannot work effectively when changes of this magnitude occur?

In addition to all the billing procedure changes, there are others that greatly affect the business operations of the practice. If you submit your charges (up to 8 on one document) according to all the new rules, if one charge rejects or pends, all others charges will also reject or pend regardless of their correctness. In other words, the payment will be delayed for an indefinite period.

The electronic submission of claims to Blue Cross-Blue Shield of Virginia guarantees increased costs for the provider. It appears that the physician(s) will be charged $150 to $250 per month plus 15 cents per claim document. This cost is in addition to any costs you've already incurred for data entry, transmission of claims via the telephone line, equipment, training, programming, etc. If, however, paper claims are submitted, there are no additional costs. But surely an influx of paper claims would cause the carrier to have increased expenses. Can you understand the rationale behind such a decision? Submitting computer-generated paper claims is an option if the computer can print all the required information.

Are other options available? You could consider using a clearing house for transmitting claims electronically, but you should be able to cost-justify your actions. A clearing house should provide you with an inquiry capability into the patient's insurance plan coverage which would be nice to have. Of course, there would be an associated cost for same, as well as a charge per line item or per document for submitting the claim electronically. Using a clearing house should also prevent claim rejections. If you don't have all the necessary information, the claim would not be processed into the system but would be returned to you for the additional information. This prevents an unusual time lag between rendering services and receiving payment. A clearing house for claim processing is an option, but it means increased costs for the physician.

In summary, it's imperative for you to keep pace with the third-party payers. Can they direct your future? It's becoming more evident that they can. Consequently, it will take skillful management, the proper automation system, the right controls for measuring your effectiveness, and the use of the "what-if" test. In addition, you need to constantly monitor possible changes. Guard yourself against irregular cash flow, claim denials, and high accounts receivable. Be prepared for the challenges of tomorrow.

7. Selecting the Software That's Best for You

Once you've decided to computerize your office, you've committed yourself to an investment of both your time and your money. Selecting an office computer system is not an easy task: You can look to others for information and direction, but the final decision is yours alone. The investment of time is vital, not only to your decision on the purchase but also to the continuing support you must provide after installation.

Preliminary Steps in Selecting a Computer System

INVESTIGATION. In the early stages, your primary concern should be to see computers in action; to see exactly what they can do. Look at various systems—both at demonstrations and in actual operation in other physicians' offices. Ask questions of computer sales representatives and customers. Don't let yourself be snowed by computer jargon—ask for plain English. You may eventually find yourself using some computer buzzwords, but you'll understand them by then.

INVOLVEMENT OF YOUR COMPUTER ADMINISTRATOR. The success or failure of your computer system will depend largely on what system you select. Input from your computer administrator is important; if possible, the selection of the person to fill this position should be made prior to choosing the computer system. Your computer administrator may have, in fact, previous experience in choosing and implementing computer systems.

PREREQUISITES. Choosing an in-house system will be much easier if you know what you *must* have, what you'd *like* to have, and what would be *nice* to have. And a basic understanding of what a computer can do is another important prerequisite.

Computer Basics

A computer is nothing more than a machine—an office machine—that can augment cerebral functions. Its speed, accuracy, and flexibility can produce a much faster turnover of accounts receivable, for example, than a manual system can. A computer doesn't replace human beings, but it does help them do their jobs better.

No matter how long you've been in practice—two, five, or 20 years—you've seen new machines or improvements in old ones that have increased efficiency in the medical office. Basically, these machines permit more work to be done in less time. The computer is just a better machine. When you compare computers to other business machines—a typewriter, for example—you can see that the difference is really a matter of degree. Both typewriters and computers speed up office procedures and increase efficiency. But a typewriter requires only muscle power to direct its use, while a computer serves to assist, augment, or replace cerebral functions (although also requiring some muscle power).

What, exactly, is a computer system? In simple terms, it is like a set of stereo components. The basic set includes the computer itself (usually in a cabinet about half the size of a standard desk, or even smaller), one or more terminals (a combination video screen and typewriter keyboard), and a printer (an electric typewriter with no keyboard).

Just as the finest stereo hardware will do nothing until an album or tape is fed into it, computer hardware needs a program of instructions (broadly called "software") to enable it to play. Software that's been specifically designed for a medical office, for example, could manage medical records, generate bills, fill out insurance forms, handle payroll, keep financial records, provide diagnostic assistance, and lots more. Different software in the same computer could monitor your stock portfolio, prepare your taxes, teach you French, or handle your word processing chores. Like a stereo, in other words, the computer plays what it's told to play.

Unlike a stereo, however, a computer won't play all by itself once it's switched on, even after the software's in place. You or your staff have to feed information into it, then order it to calculate and regurgitate the information in various forms. Feed it the list of services and procedures you performed on Mrs. Roberts, for example, then tell it to crank out a bill and a Blue Shield form—and to remember that information and everything else about Mrs. Roberts. You talk to the computer through the terminal keyboard; it responds via the terminal screen (see Fig. 7-1) and the printer.

Also unlike the stereo system, in which the equipment is more important than the albums and tapes, computer software is far more important than computer hardware. Today's state-of-the-art computer hardware, regardless of brand name, is all relatively close in quality and capability—and advanced enough to do virtually anything a medical office can ask of it. Yet doctors aren't strangers to bad computer experiences. In almost every case of a computer gone screwy, *software* is the culprit. That's why it's especially important that you understand what software is and what it can do for you.

Computer Software

Software consists of programs (sets of instructions) written in code—a special form of shorthand. It usually resides on magnetic disks. When you type instructions on the keyboard, you are "speaking" to the software. It then "speaks" to the control system (operating system), which makes the hardware perform the desired functions.

Software Categories

There are three basic categories of software: operating systems, language translators, and applications programs. While you don't need to know everything about these, a basic understanding will help you in selecting your computer system.

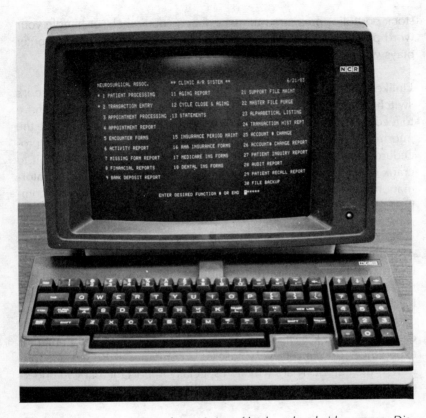

Figure 7-1. *Computer terminal, consisting of keyboard and video screen. Displayed on the screen is a typical medical-office software "menu," a listing of available functions and reports to choose from.*

OPERATING SYSTEMS. The operating system produces the communication network between computer programs and hardware. In short, it "operates" the computer so that the flow of information through it is controlled. Every modern computer has an operating system.

Major tasks of the operating system include loading applications programs into the computer, running the programs, and directing input and output. The operating system also performs such functions as sending messages to the terminal screen, checking the printer to make sure it's working correctly, and controlling the disk drives.

Your computer will come with a built-in operating system. Each manufacturer provides its own, and this usually means that various computer programs aren't directly interchangeable from one system to another without some degree of modification.

LANGUAGE TRANSLATORS. Computer languages are used to communicate instructions to the computer. Computer software packages known as translators, compilers, interpreters, or assemblers convert language statements into internal form usable by the computer. Some variety of machine language is inherent to every computer; higher-level languages were designed to make programming easier. The use of higher-level languages has led to computer systems that are more "user-friendly"—less confusing and frightening to the user.

There are three higher-level languages that you should have some familiarity with: BASIC, COBOL, and Pascal.

BASIC. BASIC stands for "Beginner's All-purpose Symbolic Instruction Code." This is about the easiest computer programming language to learn. So if you're planning on doing any programming yourself, it would be an advantage to know BASIC. One big drawback of BASIC, however, is that it is somewhat awkward to use—it's not as straightforward as might be desired. Debugging (correcting) programs can be difficult using BASIC.

COBOL. COBOL is an acronym for "COmmon Business Oriented Language." It was designed for general commercial data processing, and it is widely used in industry. The code is relatively easy to understand because of the lack of restrictions on meaningful identifying names. This reduces the need for additional documentation.

Pascal. Pascal, named after 17th-century mathematician Blaise Pascal, is a computer language designed to enhance the teaching of programming as a systematic discipline. It is a highly structured language, minimizing the possibility of programmer errors and simplifying the debugging, modification, and updating of existing programs. While Pascal is an attractive language because it is so structured, most currently available software is not written in Pascal.

APPLICATIONS PROGRAMS. Applications software requires operator input to function. These programs are designed to perform specific tasks—such as processing of accounts receivable. When computer salesmen talk about software, they're usually speaking of applications programs. You tell them a task that you want performed in your office, and they'll show you an applications program that will accomplish it.

Evaluating Your Software Needs

To properly evaluate the software you'll need—the business and medical programs that will be involved in your day-to-day operations—it's important to know exactly what your requirements are.

For example, you will be choosing between batch and on-line processing. With batch processing, all affected files are updated at the end of the function or at the end of the day. With on-line processing, all affected files are updated as information is entered by computer operators at their work stations. This provides up-to-date status information at all times—a most important feature you should consider when evaluating software for computer systems.

PREPACKAGED VERSUS CUSTOMIZED PROGRAMS. Keep in mind that you're *not* the first doctor to get a computer system. Thousands of physicians have done it before you, including, probably, doctors in your own specialty. This means that you may be able to use ready-made, prepackaged programs—literally "off the shelf"—for most of the functions that you want a computer to perform.

It's important to remember this because others—perhaps a computer salesman, perhaps another doctor—may lead you to believe that you must have custom-made programming. Custom-made programming may be appropriate to handle a function that is unique to your practice. But often it's not necessary. People often buy customized programs when they don't really know exactly what they want and need.

Customized programs can be very costly. And not only initially. If a programming error turns up days, weeks, or even months after the program is put into operation, it could cost you more money. And heaven help you if the programmer or systems analyst who designed the program isn't available. It may be impossible (or extremely expensive) for another programmer to straighten out the problem. Even regular program maintenance and support will be commensurately more expensive for a customized program than for a prepackaged one. So if at all possible, stay away from customized programs.

ADAPTABLE PREPACKAGED SOFTWARE. Another reason customized software is often unnecessary: Prepackaged programs usually have options available that will allow them to be customized to your needs. To achieve optimal results, evaluate the prepackaged medical and business programs available that will most closely meet the needs of the jobs you want done.

Adapting software to meet your needs is not only desirable, but mandatory. It's essential to know not only the needs of your practice, but also the minimal acceptable features that would be necessary in a system for your practice. All program changes are costly. It's usually better to select a more expensive prepackaged system that is designed to be adaptable than to purchase a less expensive system that will be costly to change if the need arises in the future.

USER-FRIENDLY SOFTWARE. You must also keep in mind that *people* will be operating your computer system—and they must feel comfortable with the software you choose. The more comfortable they feel, the more successful your computer operation will be. Programs are written with varying degrees of "lead-through" assistance or instructions for the computer operators. Some software is so easy to use—because the system leads the operator through it so quickly and smoothly—that training time is kept to a minimum. Errors, too, are less likely to occur with user-friendly software. This is an important feature that you shouldn't overlook.

SOFTWARE RELIABILITY. The reliability of the programming can have a large impact on the support and maintenance you receive from the vendor. This may be especially true if you go against a vendor's recommendation. Even though you purchased it from him, he's not going to want to run out to your office every few days—and the problem will be magnified if you insisted on a software program that the vendor told you might not be reliable.

COMPUTER SECURITY. A basic requirement of any software system should be security. The system should provide security for both the office and the operator. There should be controls over what an operator can and cannot do, as well as over access to the computer—entry of a security code should be required before use of a terminal for input or output is permitted.

A good security system prevents misuse of the computer. You should be able, for example, to prevent a discharged employee from erasing records. Access to the computer should be given only for specific purposes; an employee who handles, say, appointment scheduling shouldn't have access to accounts receivable. And even the accounts receivable operator should have limitations—otherwise she might give unwarranted credit to a friend or wipe out charges that should be paid to you. Specially designed software that associates certain functions and access levels with certain access codes (individually assigned to different operators) can help provide this type of security.

Judging Software Quality and Suitability

Now comes the $64,000 (which it could cost you for a computer system) question: How do you tell good software from bad? Plain and simple, good software works. If it does what it's supposed to do, not occasionally, but all the time, then it's good software.

It also has to be suited to your specific needs. Computer stores are bursting with prepackaged programs these days. A good accounts-payable program, for example, might cost you $500 or more. Inventory-control capability might run about the same amount, and general ledger another $1,000 or so. You could spend $5,000 to $10,000 for all the major programs, but you still might not have software adequate for your office.

For example, one of the most important medical-office software functions is processing of insurance forms. The computer should be able to track insurance forms, age them, amend and resubmit them, and give you reports on what's paid and what's open. Though most private carriers use standardized claim forms, Blue Shield forms differ from state to state. And until the Blues fully standardize their forms, software for your office can't be bought off a shelf ready to use. It will have to be adapted. (See Chapter 6.)

Because of that and because you'll probably need lots of maintenance support for your programs, satisfactory software is most likely to come from a vendor with a number of installations in medical offices. In addition, a national or large regional firm with strong service and programming departments is recommended.

Once you've decided what functions you want the computer to take off your hands, let the vendor show you how well his software can do them. It's no good to simply decide to computerize, then adapt your procedures to what the vendor is selling. Assuming your office is well run already, you should consider only software that will do your present procedures better—faster, more cheaply, more accurately—than you're doing them now.

What Software Can Do for You

Most consultants specializing in computerizing medical offices agree that there are three basic areas in which a computer can help: practice efficiency, financial controls, and in-depth information. While we've touched on some of these before, a quick review is in order.

PRACTICE EFFICIENCY. This means improved speed and accuracy in billing, third-party work, record-keeping, and the like. You have to take a hands-on look at several systems to get a feel for which would suit your practice best and which your staff could handle most easily. Obviously, the system should have the capability for the ICD and CPT codes to be built into it. Some systems may have these codes and the relative-value scales already built in. Another example: A directory of local ZIP codes stored in the system could save your operators a lot of time and errors.

Efficiency might also come from a step-saving program that produces a daily list of your hospital patients by room number, with the rooms arranged in order of the most convenient route through each hospital. Generally speaking, the larger your practice, the greater the efficiency improvements possible from computerizing.

FINANCIAL CONTROLS. Sometimes a computer can pay for itself just with the improvements it brings to your handling of the practice's finances. Let's say that you currently prove the posting once a month, and maybe you're consistently $500 to $1,000 off. Now you can prove by patient name every day and find the problem easily. You can also run trial balances at any time, in numeric or alphabetic order. And you can collect better: When Mrs. Roberts calls for an appointment, the system should automatically bring her balance to the screen so your receptionist can say, "And you'll be bringing a payment of $15 that day, won't you, Mrs. Roberts?"

You can also keep track of which insurance carrier owes you what and recognize an insurance problem as it's just beginning to emerge. You can break down partners' income distributions regularly, according to production, if you'd like, instead of having to deal with an unpleasant reconciliation of accounts at the end of the year.

One of the most important features that you should get from your computer system is uniform pricing for all procedures. Obviously, charges shouldn't vary among members of a group practice. However, you should still have the capability of overriding a charge when there's a reason to do so. But it should certainly be noted as an override on the computer-generated transaction report for better audit control. If you contract for discounted fee-for-service, you may need more than one uniform fee schedule, but an override should always be flagged whenever a fee is changed from the norm, no matter how many fee schedules are in place.

IN-DEPTH INFORMATION. You can learn things about your practice from your computer, too. Some systems may permit you to use that ZIP code directory, for example, to discover that most of your new patients are coming from the north end of town. Then you can analyze why and how to respond. Should you open up an office there? Affiliate with a hospital up that way? What are you doing wrong on the south side?

If Mrs. Roberts is a difficult diagnosis this time, perhaps you can get help from the data bank of patients in your vendor's entire family of doctor-clients. You can tell the computer, "Show me a list of all women, 60 or over, with arthritis in a clubfoot." If the computer produces a list of 115 and that's too many, tell it, "Okay, show me the oldest dozen." See which diagnoses compare to Mrs. Roberts's, and take clues from which diagnoses resulted in what.

Or you may be able to pull helpful information out of your own computer files to help you in diagnoses. Since all entries require a diagnosis and procedure to be entered, you should be able to get diagnosis and procedure reports. Such information as a listing of all males over 25 years of age treated for hypertension in the last six months may prove valuable.

But remember that some software packages don't allow this, while others include a medical data base that provides detailed information. Some packages provide only a total count for diagnoses treated and/or procedures performed while others may provide the total charges being generated by each procedure. You'll have to decide exactly how much information you want to know—and how much you may want in the future.

The presence of these sophisticated functions indicates a state-of-the-art system. It's also a good clue that the vendor offering it is a sophisticated software maven.

Other Software-Related Features to Consider

FLEXIBILITY. Software flexibility means several things. For example, Medicare now requires you to show the date of birth of the responsible party when you submit a claim. But at one time, that was not required. Those physicians whose software formatted files in, say, 150 characters (bytes) who didn't have room to stick in six more for date of birth needed a major—and costly—restructuring of their programs when the new requirement was announced. Built-in flexibility could have allowed for such unanticipated changes in format. (See Chapter 6.)

Flexibility can also provide the ability, for example, to change a fee, to put in a courtesy discount, or to add or delete a charge on a statement. If the mayor of your town hasn't paid you in a while, you may not want the computer to pester him with regular dunning notices.

Flexibility further means having the freedom to make certain changes in the programs yourself—adding a new doctor to the system, for example—without needing a major software service call. Or if a certain patient has three insurance coverages, you may need to bill all three companies on behalf of the patient, or you may need to bill them one at a time until you've recovered your full fee. The computer should permit you to easily accomplish such exceptions to the rule.

Ask your vendor how flexible his programs are; don't be specific, as with the date-of-birth example. Let him show you everything.

THE USER'S MANUAL. You'll also need to get a feel for the vendor's instruction manual. Can you understand it enough to solve small problems yourself? Let's say Blue Shield makes a minor change in its claim form, perhaps moving the location of the Social Security number. Will the manual tell you how to adjust for that on your printouts, or will you need an expensive service call? Somewhere in the middle of your interview with the vendor, ask a question and then say: "Hold it. Let me see if I can find that for myself in your user's manual."

The latest thing in user's manuals, which sometimes run to 1,000 pages, is to put the information right in the software itself. When you come to something you don't know how to handle, you press the question-mark key (or use some other specific question code). The software looks up that page in the manual and flashes it on the screen. Virtually the ultimate in user-friendly software, it saves your vendor big printing bucks, although it will require more disk storage space.

SOFTWARE COST. Finally, how much does medical-office software cost? It can range from about $1,000 to $35,000, and it often seems to be priced inconsistently, based on what the vendor thinks he can get for it. It does not seem to be based on his actual cost of creating it; if it were, vendor profits would probably be much lower. If you buy good software, you're probably being charged reasonably if the price is $7,000-$12,000—the middle to upper-middle range.

8. Selecting the Hardware That's Best for You

Just as with a stereo system, computer components from any of the leading manufacturers work together smoothly. Nevertheless, it's best to buy your computer and all its peripheral components from the same manufacturer. If you don't, repair service could be a problem. The printer repairman can say he's not getting a signal from the central processing unit (CPU). The CPU repairman will insist that there is a signal. And they go round and round. Meanwhile, you're left with your practice on hold.

Most experts agree that the quality of state-of-the-art hardware is fairly even from manufacturer to manufacturer today. One company may be slightly ahead in printers, while other companies may have a slight edge in CPUs, disks, or terminals. Technological advances have brought parity up and prices down, so the few bucks you'd save buying a hybrid system wouldn't be worth the maintenance headaches later on.

Since your vendor's software has probably been tailored to run on one major brand of hardware, you're probably safe in taking his recommendation. Nevertheless, you'll have to know something about the components in a system just to be able to understand a sales pitch. So here's a look at hardware:

Computer Hardware Basics

That storage disk mentioned earlier is the computer equivalent of file space; it's where the information you feed the computer actually goes. The disk is circular and magnetic; a number of disk platters are packaged together in a hard plastic case; the platters and case are called a disk pack. Disk packs are often portable, but when in use, the pack and its power device, the disk drive, usually reside inside the main computer unit. If you have a very large system, the disk will have a separate cabinet of its own.

The main unit is called the central processing unit, or CPU. The CPU also contains its own memory, sometimes referred to as core memory. Although originally called that because it consisted of magnetic cores, today's "core" memory is often in the form of semiconductor integrated circuits. One way to measure computer power is in terms of the size of the chips holding the circuits. Personal computers (like the smallest Apples, Radio Shacks, and Commodores) shouldn't be considered for your practice because the chips are too small. They don't have sufficient power and memory for most medical-office applications.

The CPU is composed of three parts: the control unit, the arithmetic unit, and the storage unit.

The control unit monitors the execution of instructions that are given to the machine. These predetermined sets of instructions constitute programs. Consequently, the control unit assures that programs are performed in proper sequence. It also coordinates input and output.

The arithmetic unit actually performs the adding, subtracting, multiplying, and dividing. These operations are handled by electronic circuits. Since there are no moving parts in the calculating process, the arithmetic is performed at almost the speed of light.

The storage unit is the memory section of the CPU. The program is stored in the memory during its execution, along with the instructions for carrying it out. The control unit activates the memory, assures the performance of the arithmetic unit, and, when necessary, activates the input and output equipment.

Other components include terminals, through which you and the computer communicate (Fig. 8-1), and printers, through which the system spews forth forms and reports. Unlike a stereo system, for which you don't need a tape deck if you don't want one, you'll need all these items before you actually have a computer system.

How to Decide What Hardware to Buy

THE CPU. In buying your CPU—the basic computer unit—there aren't a lot of decisions to make, but there are three major questions that you should be sure your vendor answers knowledgeably.

1. Are you limited by this CPU? Specifically, how much core memory and how much disk storage can you add to it? If you have 64,000 bytes (64K) of core memory (a relatively small amount), that may be enough for you now. But can it be upgraded to 128K or 512K if your practice expands, or if you take in more partners, of if you increase your disk capacity, or if you decide to add extra terminals?

The exact amount of memory you need right now could vary from vendor to vendor. If one specifies 256K and another 512K, both could be steering you straight. One might have software more complex than the other's; one might specify four terminals for your office instead of three; yet another might just want to be safe. If you have a small practice, though, and your vendor recommends a small amount of disk storage and a large amount of core memory, it could indicate that his software is sloppily written and needs a lot of CPU memory to make it perform.

Core memory manages the disk. If you have a large amount of disk storage with lots of information crammed onto it, you need a correspondingly large amount of core memory to find and retrieve that information. Your computer should respond in three seconds or less to anything you ask of it; insufficient core memory laboring under lots of

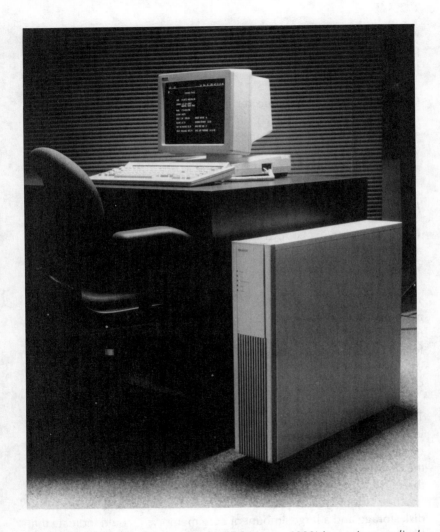

Figure 8-1. A typical minicomputer (ADDS Mentor 6000) in use in a medical office. This system includes two printers—a line printer, which uses the same stock paper for nearly all types of reports, and a matrix printer, which is continuously loaded with paper specially formatted for demand statements. The use of two printers prevents frequent, time-consuming changing of paper stock.

disk storage could take 15 to 40 seconds just to find a file. Since sufficient core memory makes the machine faster and adding more is only moderately more expensive, you might as well specify plenty.

2. How much additional disk storage should you allow for? That will help determine how big your practice can get before you need a new, larger CPU. If you're currently in a small partnership, but you envision eventual growth to a 10-doctor group, you might as well buy a CPU with the ultimate capacity for that size practice.

Trade-in or resale value on less-than-state-of-the-art hardware (which today's new equipment will be in a relatively short time) is very low.

3. How many terminals can the CPU handle, how many can it expand to, and will it allow all of them to be used at once? One of the most important features is whether or not the computer has the capability of multiprogramming—executing two or more programs during the same time period. If Sally is doing posting, can Jane enter a new patient on another terminal? When Mrs. Jones asks for her bill, does one of them have to stop? Or can Mary get on a third terminal and take care of Mrs. Jones? Can reports be printed out while other data are being entered?

Some systems can handle only one job at a time. Obviously, this can hinder your whole office operation. But many CPUs allow several jobs to be performed at once. In evaluating CPUs, it's important to know whether the system can support your demands.

In short, don't let your practice be limited in any way by your CPU.

DISK STORAGE. How much disk storage space do you need? Probably less than you think, but the rule of thumb is to buy at least twice what you currently require. The cost curve on disk drives is such that to buy a lot more is only slightly more expensive, making it foolish to be under-disked.

Disks may be rigid or of flexible Mylar material. The flexible disks are known as diskettes, floppy disks, or just "floppies." Diskettes are enclosed in an envelope with a slot for the read/write head, and can be interchanged to increase the storage capacity of each diskette drive unit. Hard disks are far more costly than diskettes but have much greater storage capacity.

Disk space is measured in megabytes. Ten megabytes of disk space, for example, can hold 10 million characters (or typewriter strokes) of information. That's roughly enough storage space for a typical surgical practice to keep records on 2,000 patients and not run out of room for 15 months or so. Disk technology comes in a wide range of capacities and costs. As technology continues to improve disk density—the amount of information that can be stored in the same amount of disk space—disk cost per megabyte becomes more affordable.

Your specialty influences the amount of disk capacity you'll need. If you're an internist, you probably perform several more services per typical patient than a surgeon does, and you might see 10 or more patients to his one. Each patient is a bill, and each service is a line item on a bill, so you need more disk space than a surgeon (with a comparable practice) does. If you're a family practitioner, you'll want to keep records in the computer for 15, 18, 24 or more months; a year and a half from now, Mrs. Jones might ask how much she paid you last year.

So the amount of disk storage you need can vary depending on your specialty and business volume. The software vendor should be the one to decide how much that amounts to. Your job is simply to tell him the nature of your practice, how much detail you want to keep, and for how long.

Unfortunately, this is where an unscrupulous vendor can sandbag the unwitting doctor. One of the biggest abuses in the computer business is to "lowball" the customer on disk storage, just to keep the total price down and get the sale. The user then goes six months with a small disk capacity and runs out of space. The vendor comes back and sells him what he really needed in the first place. Often this involves de-installation, re-installation, software conversion, and, of course, lots more money. Some vendors line their pockets this way.

The only way to protect yourself is to ask the vendor if he's selling you a big enough system to handle your practice as you described it to him, in the amount of detail you want your records to hold, for the time period you want to keep them. Then tell him you want an addendum to the sales contract specifying that he'll take back your system and apply its remaining value—prorated over five years—to the cost of a larger one, if it turns out you needed more than you were sold.

Regardless of how much disk storage you buy, you'll eventually fill it up. You'll know you're getting close to capacity when the computer's response time begins to lengthen. A keyboard command that used to bring a response in two or three seconds now takes 30 to 45 seconds or more. At that point, you'll have to either add more disk capacity or, more likely, purge some of your present disk storage.

Purging is the computer equivalent of carrying old files down to the basement. Your vendor should give you the ability to selectively remove old data from the disk by copying it onto a tape that you can then store permanently in some safe place. Tell him how you'd like to do it: Perhaps every month you'll remove at least the detail from all patient files that have had no activity—and no outstanding balance—for 15 months. You might not wish to remove the demographic data—name, address, date of birth, etc.—just the service detail. You might also leave your "comments" information and "last diagnosis."

With the price of disk capacity falling rapidly, doctors will have the capability to store much more information very economically. In the future, the need to purge will probably be much less frequent.

THE TERMINALS. They come in a thousand styles, and you can spend from a few hundred to a few thousand dollars on one. At the low end, you'll get a keyboard with a couple of wires for hooking up to your own television. At the high end, you'll get a sophisticated, stylish terminal with intelligence of its own built in—self-contained memory that might allow you to edit without going through the CPU, for example. Don't bother with terminals at either extreme.

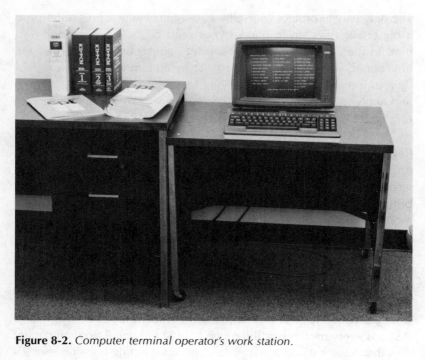

Figure 8-2. Computer terminal operator's work station.

You can probably get just what you need for less than $500. You don't want the most sophisticated, complex terminal on the market; you want the simplest one that will work for you. Operators should be given the least possible opportunity to make data-entry errors, and a keyboard full of hieroglyphics is just asking for trouble.

One vendor, who color-codes his keyboards for the sake of simplicity, tells of a gadget-freak doctor who demanded the most sophisticated keyboard he could find. It took the doctor two weeks to teach the system to his assistant, and then he had to pay her more money. "I'm a computer operator now," she claimed. A benchmark to keep in mind when choosing terminals: The slowest learner on your staff should be able to master it in four hours.

The number of terminals you'll need is based on the volume of business you do and the speed of your operators. In general, if your practice sees 50 to 100 patients a day, performing an average of two services on each, you'll need one terminal. (But note that the advantages of multiprogramming—discussed in Chapter 12—are lost when you have only one terminal.) If you see 75 patients a day but do five services each time, you'll need two. If it's 125 patients and two services, you'll need 1.25 terminals—in which case you should buy two. Considering the system's overall cost, an extra terminal is a small extra expense. And a basic rule is *never* to let your computer limit you. If it's one of your operators who's holding you back, though, you'll have to discharge or reassign her.

Terminal screens come in amber, green, or gray. No study has conclusively proved which color is easiest on the eyes. It is certain, however, that a full-color screen is unnecessary—and an added maintenance problem that you can do without.

THE PRINTER. Because they're electromechanical devices, printers are far more prone to breakdowns and failures than such all-electronic devices as CPUs. Printers are classified by speeds, ranging from 30 characters per second up to 1,200 lines per minute. Generally, slower printers are more reliable, while faster ones have higher maintenance costs and shorter stretches between failures. Choosing one is a trade-off between enough speed to get your work done, but not so much that your system is frequently down for printer maintenance. The average time between breakdowns for printers of all speeds is only eight to nine months.

So how fast a printer do you need and how much should it cost? A 30-character-per-second printer will do for anything from a solo practitioner up to, perhaps, a low-volume three-doctor practice. The cost can range from $800 or so for a cheap, off-brand model up to around $3,000. A better choice for a solo practice or small group, though, might be a major-brand 150-line-per-minute printer that you can pick up for about $4,000. The 300 lpm will cost $6,000 and up; and 600 lpm will cost $9,000 and up. But some microcomputers cannot handle such fast printers.

If your office uses cycle billing or some other method of spreading the work over the whole month—if you don't need to print all your bills and insurance forms in one day—you probably don't need a high-speed printer at all. One management consultant, in fact, says that he never advises more than a 200-lpm printer for a doctor. He feels that even for a 40-doctor group, two or three medium-speed printers are better than one 1,000-lpm headache.

The breakdown problem can be crippling. Many computer systems shut down entirely when the printer goes out of action. To safeguard your office from being hostage to a flaky printer, ask your vendor for "spooler" capability, a software feature. Spooling sets aside a place on the disk for the computer to put the work it's done—to "print" on the disk, so to speak—until your temperamental printer feels like working again. Then when the printer's fixed, spooler capability will allow your system to print reports in any job sequence, instead of being locked into printing them in the order they were entered. If, for example, you've just entered data for 500 third-party forms when Mrs. Roberts asks for a copy of her last bill, spooler capability will let you take care of her first. The claims data can wait on the disk.

With printer breakdowns so frequent, you should also insist that your vendor provide self-test capability with your printer. If your system does shut down, the printer is where you begin troubleshooting. With the self-test feature, you can order the printer—independent of the rest of the system—to print out every character it has, thereby telling you whether your current problem is with the printer.

Also make sure that your printer is wired directly to the CPU, and not through a terminal. Wiring it through a terminal is cheaper for the vendor, but it slows down the printer dramatically (by half or more) and can create printer traffic problems.

If your practice is large enough to justify more than one printer, and if your software allows you to do basic word processing, you might consider giving the second printer the capability of being upgraded from dot-matrix printing (what you might think of as a typical computer typeface) to near-letter-quality printing. For a medium-sized printer from a major manufacturer, the upgrading may involve just inserting an extra circuit board. Although a stand-alone word processing system is usually best for your practice's major letters (see Chapter 2), your computer system may be able to handle regular, smaller communications and notices. Such items as patient recall letters, collection letters to be generated as accounts age, and thank-you notes for referrals do not take up much disk space and may be appropriate to create and print using your office computer.

There are two types of printers you absolutely don't want for heavy-duty use: a daisy-wheel printer (good for letter-quality work but very slow *and* a maintenance nightmare) or a thermal printer (very inexpensive, but unable to print multiple copies).

Computerizing your office is such a major move that you should proceed with the utmost caution. Buying equipment is, like the old song says about love, where "fools rush in where angels fear to tread." Proceed only after careful investigation and acquisition of the best advice you can find.

9. Preparing to Shop for Your Computer System

In the last two chapters, we discussed in detail how you should choose the software and equipment for your computer system. But there's more—much more—than just selecting the hardware, software, and peripherals that will do the job that you want done in your office. You also have to know how to shop for this equipment.

Shopping strategy isn't just price, either: You don't do it the way you purchase a car—by visiting several dealers and trying to get the best bottom-line figure. If something goes wrong on the car, you just bring it in for service. If the dealer's service department isn't as good as you think it should be, you can complain to the manufacturer. And if the car's just a lemon, you can sell it and buy something else with not a lot of inconvenience.

But if you buy a computer that's a lemon, or the dealer has a lousy service department, it could cost you all kinds of grief—and a ton of money. And even if you buy a good computer from a reliable dealer, you could soon find yourself with a dinosaur because of the rapidly changing technology in the computer field.

How, then, do you become a careful computer shopper? The best way is to develop a clear idea of what you want to accomplish and to pursue a cautious, step-by-step approach. Here are the basic eight steps to take:

Step 1: Know What's Different About Your Practice

If you're practicing pediatrics, say, the length of time patients must stay in your data base would be entirely different from that of a general surgeon. Other examples: The parents or guardians are the responsible parties, not the patient. Last names (patient and parents) are often different. You treat childhood diseases. You provide immunizations routinely. You're a primary care physician. A uniform per capita payment or fee does—or can—affect you. You have four satellite offices. Gross receipts must be maintained by location for tax purposes. You need to know whether or not each location is profitable.

If you practice general surgery, your procedures would be different. Seventy-five percent of your patients may have Medicare insurance. You must have a census sheet for hospital patients to do your rounding. You have contracted with a plan carrier for discounted fee-for-service. You write articles for publication. You need to know the physicians who refer to you.

Make your list as extensive as possible.

Step 2: Know What's Not Different About Your Practice

Medicine differs from other businesses, mainly because of confidentiality and the very nature of the transactions. This is the primary reason you need to deal with a vendor who has expertise in the health-care field.

Skills between the physicians and their staffs are vastly different. The complexities of practicing medicine may require a sophisticated program to serve your needs, but it also requires one that is user-friendly and simple to use.

The practice structure is basically the same for all physicians—either solo, group, or clinic.

You're a primary care physician or a specialist.

Your accounting, claim-processing, and billing needs are about the same.

By now you're probably getting the idea that what works for one practice may not work for another practice, and you're exactly right. The needs for primary care physicians are different from those of a specialist, and the needs for primary care physicians differ between OB-GYN, family practice, and pediatrics. Specialists' needs also are quite different between specialties. Recognizing similarities, however, should reduce the time you spend investigating systems.

The system you select must work for your practice. The best advice will come from physicians with practices like yours, i.e., the same specialty and similar patient loads. You don't need a degree in computer science to buy a computer, but you do need some familiarity with the marketplace. Always consult with other doctors who have computerized.

Step 3: Complete an Evaluation of Your Business Operations

How is everything currently being done? To assess the organization and efficiency of your business operations and office procedures, you must know how your current system operates. If you don't know the reason for every piece of paper and how it's handled by your staff—and for what purposes—how could you possibly evaluate whether or not a computer system would be adaptable to your practice? Another reason this step is so important is that a computer system must work for you; your staff should never have to work for a computer!

The easiest way to start is to secure a sample of every form used in your practice and then examine each form in detail.

NEW PATIENT REGISTRATION FORM. Are you obtaining all the necessary information to collect the account? Do you know not only the patient's employer and address but also the spouse's? Do you know the name, address, telephone number, and relationship of the closest relative (not spouse)? Do you know who referred the patient? Is your insurance information adequate? Do you know the primary and secondary insurance carrier, and do you have their addresses for mailing the claims? Do you have space on this form for assigning account numbers and for recording authorization numbers? (The authorization number is provided by a primary care physician in a HMO setting, authorizing you to see the patient for a specified number of visits, quite often only one.) Do you obtain a signed authorization for release of information, as necessary to process insurance claims, and also for assigning the benefits payable to you? Does it state that a photocopy of the authorization and assignment will be considered as valid as the original?

Are you beginning to see that although medicine is not a business, there is business in medicine?

Will the computer you select be able to store all the patient information data? Probably not! It will store the data pertinent to billing. It may be necessary to continue having your patients complete a registration form and obtain photocopies of insurance cards, but computer registration should still not take more than one minute.

An evaluation also may prove that you're currently not obtaining enough information from the patient to collect the account. The need for redesigning your new patient registration form may become evident, but also keep in mind that a computer may cause you to redesign the form also, since the information on the form should flow in the exact order as required by the computer.

EXAMINE YOUR FEE SLIP. Know who handles it and for what purposes. Are the patient's next appointment and/or the medications you prescribed recorded on it? Is it prenumbered? Can mathematical error occur when pricing procedures?

A good computer system can generate prenumbered encounter forms (fee slips) and should give you better control. It will provide uniform pricing and do all the financial calculations. If the patient's next appointment is keyed into the system, you should be able to recall those patients who did not keep their scheduled appointments, as well as send a letter to them for failure to abide by your instructions. This could significantly reduce a liability claim's ever getting into court; in fact, you may have a counter-suit, contributory negligence on the part of the patient.

If the system allows for keying in your prescribed medications, a simple command should produce a listing, for example, of the patients you have placed on a drug that has been recalled. The search should be quick and effortless. Computers can also generate how drugs should be taken and/or what any adverse reactions might be, but it's all dependent upon your needs and the system you select.

The nature of the information entered into a computer for registering and billing a patient should allow a data base for retrieving the information if you need it. But don't count on it. You need to know what the system can and cannot do for you.

Knowing who handles the paper in your office—and for what purpose—will help you determine who will be affected by a computer system and to what extent.

Step 4: Determine Your Needs

Make a list for (1) must have, (2) like to have, and (3) nice to have. For example, you must have a computer that will do your accounting, process insurance claims, and generate bills. But you would like to have a computer that has a data base for retrieving clinical information, and it would be nice to have a word processor.

The vendor will price your computer accordingly. You may find you need to give up a "nice to have" or "like to have" to implement a "must have." You may also find that there are more costs associated with your "must have" than you had expected. The lists, no doubt, will help you determine trade-offs, i.e., giving up one requirement to institute another. It will also help you to recognize what a computer can and cannot do for your practice.

Step 5: What Changes Are Necessary to Accommodate This Technology?

If problems currently exist, they must be identified and solutions sought prior to any installation and implementation of a computer system. If a medical office is in chaos now, a computer system would only serve to compound the problems.

Site changes are necessary for a computer system. Environmental controls are essential. Excessive temperatures—hot or cold—may play havoc on some systems, as will dust. Many computers have had unnecessary downtime from coffee being accidentally spilled into the system or paper clips falling into keyboards. Static electricity also can cause unnecessary downtime.

CPUs often need a dedicated, insulated, and isolated 220 or 110 power line. Peripheral equipment—printers and CRTs—may need special lines or may not be able to share line use with other heavy equipment. Telephone modems also require installation.

To accommodate the new technology, you'll probably find that there's a need to reorganize the assignment of staff duties. This, however, should be an assignment for the computer administrator and not take away from the doctors' productivity time.

You will no doubt find that your forms and statements will have to be redesigned for a computer. In addition, your evaluation should prove that indeed you're going to need leadership to bring about the change—to take you from a manual system or an inadequate computer system to a computerized system that will handle your requirements.

Being prepared for all the changes that will occur with the new technology should help ensure a smooth transition and successful implementation. This step should never be overlooked.

Step 6: What Can Be Done Better with a Computer?

Write down your expectations or objectives for getting a computer system. Many doctors have been disappointed because they selected a system that would not do what they thought it would. For example, suppose you need a daily hospital rounding list. Will the system generate it? Yes! But the way it's done by the computer may not be what you need. If you're in a group practice, the computer may generate a listing of all patients in each hospital by doctor, but it may not be able to generate a combined listing of all patients per hospital. If there are seven physicians in your group and you're on first call for weekend coverage, it would mean that you would have to look in seven different places on the rounding schedule to make sure you had seen all the patients on one floor in one hospital. If you cover multiple floors within the hospital and also multiple hospitals, this procedure may not work for you. You may revert to your manual system again and then have to pay for costly program changes.

If you write down your expectations now, you'll find yourself becoming more explicit as your knowledge increases relative to computerizing your medical offices. You'll also be better prepared to state your objectives in your request for proposal (RFP). (See Chapter 10.)

Step 7: Know How the Computer Will Affect Your Staff

Job descriptions will change, and you'll only want to involve your personnel to the extent of how the computer will affect each one individually. The ones who will be doing data processing will be more involved than the ones who will only use inquiry to answer patients' questions about their accounts.

Step 8: Know Your Practice Characteristics and Be Able to Project Your Growth

You'll need to provide the vendor with statistical information about your practice, such as how many active patients you have, how many monthly statements you mail, how many transactions you post per patient, etc. An in-depth practice analysis must be completed before you can shop for a system.

The analysis should allow you to determine what you'll currently need a computer to do for you. A mandatory requirement might be that you need a system that will do your accounts receivable, insurance claim processing and billing, and one that has communication capabilities.

To help ensure that you get a system that can grow with the practice, you'll need to project the future growth of the practice within a given time frame, and project the computer applications that you'll be adding to the system. For example, within three years you'll be adding two physicians and your active accounts will increase to "X" (how many?). You also expect to add word processing to the system by the end of the second year and medical records by the end of the fourth year. The vendor will determine the system you need based upon the information you provide.

In summary, there are no short cuts for selecting the right computer for your practice. It takes work on your part. You need a culmination of knowledge about your practice and the patients you serve. In addition, there is still more homework to accomplish!

READ UP. If you think you can get away with a small computer system, scan the ads in business publications, the *Wall Street Journal*, and the numerous computer magazines sold on newsstands. This will give you an idea of what's available and the kind of performance (e.g., amount of memory, printer speed, number of characters that can be displayed on the video screen) that you can expect for your money.

ATTEND SEMINARS. A number of computer firms offer free, one-day seminars for the computer novice. These sessions, of course, include an obligatory—though usually low-key—sales pitch, but they can provide a good primer on computer use. Some of these seminars may be devoted exclusively to medical applications. It's probably a good idea to have your computer administrator (and your office manager if she's not the administrator) attend the sessions with you and help evaluate the machines in relation to your practice's problems.

TRY A HOBBYIST'S SETUP. If you're really gung-ho, consider investing in an inexpensive personal computer. One pediatrician purchased a small Radio Shack machine "so I could find out something about programming and learn the right questions to ask when I went shopping for a system for my practice." And a cardiologist bought a little Heathkit training computer that "helped me immensely." (But be aware that the data stored by your small computer will probably *not* be directly transferable into any large system.)

Purchasing a personal computer represents a relatively low-cost introduction to recreational data processing. When you outgrow the system, you can give it to your children.

10. Shopping Strategy— The RFP

If you're thinking of buying an inexpensive personal computer, you don't need an RFP, or "request for proposal." But for more costly or more sophisticated equipment, an RFP is an important shopping tool.

An RFP is nothing more than an invitation to prospective suppliers. You tell them what problems you want solved or what you want in the way of equipment, and invite them to submit bids to supply you with a system.

What to Include

Specific requirements and any conditions you expect the vendor to meet should be spelled out in the RFP. It should also include a detailed analysis of the paperwork and record-keeping performed in your office—e.g., the number of Medicare and other third-party claims you handle, the number of patient statements you mail, and so forth. Finally, it should spell out your basic objectives in buying a computer—e.g., to expedite the processing of insurance forms, to improve collections on accounts more than 30 days overdue, and the like.

The more details you can provide about your practice, the better. Be equally specific in listing your needs and objectives. For example, you may want to reduce the time you spend processing bills every month from three days to one. To meet this objective, you need assurance that a vendor can supply you with timely service in case the computer breaks down. To get that assurance, you need to state in the RFP that the vendor must respond to a service call within a specified number of hours. Otherwise you may miss your billing deadline if a computer problem develops.

Who Should Help You

Your computer administrator should, with your input, be able to draw up an RFP. You may also want to bring in an outside consultant to help you produce one. Some doctors have used their accounting firms to assist them in preparing RFPs.

The advantage of going through this exercise, at the very least, is that an RFP will force you to take a careful look at how your office functions. It will force vendors to respond in a common format, thereby making it easier for you to compare their offerings. It will enable you, the vendor, and your computer administrator to identify and examine certain trade-offs. You may, for example, find that you can get by with a slower but less expensive printer if you're willing to devote an extra day to processing bills.

An RFP may be extremely simple (Table 10-1) or detailed. The more details that you provide the greater the likelihood that the computer you select will work for you. Assuming that you're prepared to shop for a computer system (Chapter 9), we'll delve into the RFP.

Study Table 10-1. Could you complete this RFP accurately at this very moment? Do you know your present practice characteristics? This information is vital! Have you thought about your future growth? You do need to project it if you plan to select a system that will grow with you.

Look at the table again. Does it tell the vendor that you must be able to produce a single statement on demand and, in addition, that the program must allow for cycle billing? Or that you need the ability to display the primary and secondary insurance carriers on the claim form, inverting their position on the second insurance claim?

Do you see how you could select a computer system, have it installed and implemented, and then find out it can't do what you expected it to do? This has happened to many physicians. Is it the vendor's fault? No! The physicians probably have attended computer demonstrations and possibly have seen systems in operation in a colleague's office but never thought to seek out this type of information. They took for granted that the system would do whatever was necessary for their practice. If only they had involved their personnel, someone may have recognized that this system would not work without modification or program changes.

Although Table 10-1 provides you with the basic information the vendors will need, it does not provide the details needed to select the best possible system for your practice. Let's take a look at more specifics.

ACCOUNT NUMBERS (SELECT ONE). (1) System must provide account numbers automatically; or (2) it must maintain current account numbering system in use and special requirements are as follows. (List special requirements.)

With a computer every account must have a number. It does not mean you must begin filing numerically. It does demonstrate that you need to access computer files by patient name or number. You also may have a need for referencing files by guarantor's name.

Some systems will allow you to enter a couple of alpha characters— say, the first two in the last name—and will provide you with a listing of all names starting with those letters, including the account number, address, policy number, date of birth, etc. This is an excellent feature, particularly if you have forgotten how to spell the last name or you simply cannot read someone else's handwriting. If you have several patients by the same name, it will help you identify the correct account. But don't assume all systems have this capability. With some programs, if you don't spell the name exactly as it was entered into the

Table 10-1. *Simple Request for Proposal—Family Practice*

Practice characteristics	Present	Planned growth In 5 years
Number of physicians	2	4
Number of office locations	3	5
Number of active patient charts	1,400	28,000
Number of inactive patient charts	1,200	18,000
Annual new patients	550	1,100
Annual deleted patients	300	600
Patient office visits per day	120	300
Patient hospital visits per day	30	50
Procedures per patient visit	3	3
Diagnoses per patient visit	2	3
Medications per patient visit	2	2
Total charges per day	150	350
Total payments per day	140	320
Total adjustments per day	70	250
Patient file inquiries per day	100	200
Statements per month	700	500
Insurance forms per month	400	1,000
In-house lab tests per month	1,200	1,600
In-house x-ray exams per month	1,200	1,600
In-house ECG exams per month	40	60

Applications to be implemented	Present mandatory	Planned mandatory growth in 5 years
Patient billing/accounts receivable	X	
Medical records		X
Word processing		X
Appointments and scheduling	X	
Payroll		X
Accounts payable		X
General ledger		X
Cost accounting		X
Inventory control		X
Management and marketing		X
Research		X
Communications capability	X	
Concurrent users expected	2	5
Keyboard/display units required (80-character by 24-line display capacity)	3	6
Letter quality printer	1	1
Line printer (100 LPM)	1	1

computer—even if it was misspelled—you will not get any help from the computer.

It may be advantageous to have the computer assign account numbers to new accounts. It will eliminate staff work, and their extra time can be used more productively. If you currently have a good numeric system in place, however, you may not want to change it. Don't assume that your numeric system will be unaffected by a computer. For example, suppose you use two alpha characters (the first two characters of the last name or two characters identifying the primary insurance carrier) followed by numbers as the basis for your account numbering system, the computer may not allow for the entering of alpha characters, or if you're using eight digits for your account number, the computer may only support six digits.

Let's say you prefer to keep your current numeric system. By providing the vendors with this information, they can determine whether or not they can accommodate your need or what it would cost to modify the program for you. Of course, in all probability you'll have to pay the cost for modification.

Now a decision must be made. Is it worth the cost or should the numeric system be placed in the category of "what changes are necessary to accommodate this technology" (Chapter 9, Step 5)? If it's more feasible to change your numeric system, at least, you'll be prepared for it.

Don't assume that all systems generate account numbers automatically. Ask, does it? Better yet, put it in your RFP.

FINANCIAL CLASSIFICATIONS. Although terminology may vary between vendors, you need a system that will track productivity for enhancing your knowledge about your business operations. Although you need to know the amount charged per procedure performed on a month-to-date and year-to-date basis, it also may be helpful to know the total amount charged for laboratory work, for example, rather than receiving a total for hemoglobin, another total for urinalysis, another for CBC, etc. In order to accomplish this, however, each procedure is assigned a financial classification or department, providing you a more in-depth report. Do you need a system that will summarize your charges into categories, or will a system that provides detailed financial information according to procedure performed be sufficient? Is there an option available? If so, make the computer work for you and state your need in the RFP.

PAYMENT CENTERS. Where does your money come from? In most offices there is a need to know. Can you categorize payments—for example, cash, personal check, money order, Blue Shield, Medicare, Medicaid, and by each commercial carrier and/or HMO, PPO, IPA that may be beneficial to you? Even though a program may allow flexibility, it may also have limitations. If you need 25 payment centers and the system only allows for 15, you have a problem. There are restrictions in every area, and you need to know how the restrictions can affect you.

ADJUSTMENT CODES. Because of the major changes occurring in the practice of medicine and billing procedures, adjustments to your accounts receivable need to be recorded in detail. Many systems give you the option of doing "the" write-off when payment is posted. Your accounts receivable will remain accurate, but you'll never know why! Be explicit in defining your write-offs. In the past, you could get by with a few, but today you need to know what is being written off caused by your participation in various plans offered by third-party payers: the difference between your charge and the allowed charge. For example, classify these reductions for Blue Shield, Medicare, Medicaid, etc. There also may be a need for "doctors' write-off" and "professional courtesy." Other write-off groupings may include charity, bad debt, account to collector, and risk factors according to specific plans. What's the maximum number of adjustment codes allowed by the program?

NUMBER OF PHYSICIANS IN GROUP AND NUMBER OF OFFICE LOCATIONS. Although you can quickly provide this information, how many office locations will the system support? How many physicians? Do you need to track procedures performed, adjustments to accounts, and revenue received by doctor, by office location? Is there also a need for summarizing the information into a report combining all locations by doctor? The vendor needs to know what you need.

PROCEDURE CODES AND FEES. It's essential to build your fee schedule by CPT codes, but do you also need to do it by any other coding system? Do you need more than one fee schedule? Have you entered into any contracts for discounted fee-for-service? Do you have the ability to add or delete procedure codes and/or change your fee schedule, or is this only done by the vendor?

DIAGNOSES. Do you need any coding system other than the ICD? Is there a need to record more than one diagnosis per procedure performed?

TRANSACTIONS. List your requirements, such as:

1. Charges, adjustments, and payments must be posted by physician and by office location.
2. We want the ability to override a charge but have the system flag it in the audit trail.
3. Payments are to be posted to the transaction (or you may prefer to open balance).

INSURANCE CLAIM PROCESSING. What are your requirements? What type of insurance do you process now, or in what insurance plans are your patients enrolled? Are special claim forms required? Do you complete disability claims? Are you interested in submitting paperless claims? Do you want the address of the insurance company to print on the copies? (See Chapter 11.)

BILLING. You'll probably want to have the ability to render statements on demand, as well as to render itemized statements on a regular monthly basis. After a statement has been itemized, a balance forward should be entered on the patient's next bill but with itemization of services occurring after the last billing date; however, if a total itemization should be necessary, such as at the end of the calendar year for tax purposes or simply as requested by the patient, the ability to render the statement is essential. You do not want total itemization from the time the patient was initially seen to present on every regular monthly statement rendered. This could result in the statement being so long that it could cost you several dollars to mail.

With a computer, it is advantageous to do cycle billing rather than billing all patients on the same day each month. Do you want to cycle bills on a daily basis? Weekly basis? Do you need to cycle-bill numerically? Alphabetically? Would you prefer to cycle-bill by any other method?

Do you want to do family billing or individual billing?

The vendor needs to know all special billing requirements. Other considerations may include:

1. Statements are to be printed by zip code sequence for postal savings.
2. Patient's full name must be printed on all statements when different from guarantor's name.
3. Messages are to be printed as account balance ages.
4. Collection letters are to be computer-generated.
5. Data mailers (self-contained statements with return envelopes) will be used.

ENCOUNTER FORMS OR FEE SLIPS. Forms are to be computer-generated and prenumbered for tracking.

ACCOUNTS RECEIVABLE INQUIRY. Can a search be accomplished by patient's name, guarantor's name, and account number? Will the system allow for a search by entering the first two alpha characters of the patient's last name: for instance, BR? Will it display all patients whose last name starts with BR? When doing an inquiry will the operator need to see the demographic information, as well as the detailed transactions? Will the program accommodate your needs?

PURGING ACCOUNTS. How are the accounts purged? Can you specify that all transactions that have a zero balance older than 18 months be purged but keep the demographics in the system? You may want to purge all accounts, including demographics, that have had a zero balance for six months or more, or all accounts when a zero balance occurs. Will the system allow for selectivity?

REPORTS. All the reports in the system have been designed by computer people; you probably don't need all of them. What would be useful to you? The following suggestions may help get you started:

1. Detailed financial reports by doctors, by office locations, and group summary by doctor for all locations.
2. Daily audit reports, ensuring that the system is in balance or, if out of balance, flagging the daily activities. Report should include daily totals for charges, adjustments, and payments, as well as month-to-date and year-to-date totals.
3. Financial report by procedures performed and summary report by financial classifications or departments.
4. Physician referral report.
5. Accounts receivable aging analysis extended to "X" days and beyond.
6. Reports for selectively retrieving account balance.
7. Report for "no bill" accounts.
8. Data base reporting for _____.

ACCOUNTS RECEIVABLE AGING ANALYSIS. This report is an excellent resource for working the accounts and increasing collections. All the collection clerk should need is the report and the telephone to accomplish her work. Does the report contain sufficient information? For example, John Doe owes you $150; $100 is current and $50 is 120 days old. Does the report provide the date of the last payment? Would that date affect whether or not the patient should be contacted? Does the report identify the patient's pay code, such as self-pay, Medicare, Medicaid, etc.? The staff needs to know who they can and cannot call.

The report should also provide you with detailed financial information about your accounts, i.e., dollar totals and percentages with each aging category and the grand total of your accounts receivable.

Some programs age accounts to 90 days and beyond, whereas other programs may extend the aging up to 180 days and beyond. What would be the requirement for your practice?

Will the system allow you to selectively retrieve data relative to account balances? Can you obtain a listing of accounts over 90 days old with a balance of $300 or more? A listing of all accounts billed to Medicaid with a remaining balance?

SYSTEM SECURITY. Security may range from basically nothing (one password for everyone) to comprehensive. You need adequate protection and you, at least, must have adequate control. Since the information on the computer is confidential, you must abide by privacy constraints.

The backup media provides security for you should anything happen to the computer. But have you stopped for a moment to think that if the backup media were stolen, even if it was not current, someone would have access to all your files through a given date, and you could be held liable, particularly if the proper precautions for security had not been enforced?

What type of security does the system provide? How is the security controlled? Where will you store the backup media? Who will be responsible for it?

Security may be costly, but not having it or implementing it can be far more costly.

EXPECTATIONS. If you'll write down your expectations, it will help ensure that nothing is overlooked or will reinforce some of your decisions. Examples follow:

1. Computer administrator/operator can access diagnosis and procedure files to add or delete same or to change a fee by a special security password.
2. The description for procedure will print on the insurance claim and

the patient's statement, but the diagnosis will only print on the insurance claim.

3. If insurance format changes, it will not require an expensive program change.
4. The vendor will respond to a service call within one hour and will be on site, if necessary, within four hours.
5. Within 24 months, appointment scheduling will be added to the system.

OBJECTIVES. What do you want the system to achieve? Put it down in black and white. You should be able to measure your success by your objectives. All you need to do is ask, "Have we succeeded?"

Note: Not to specify objectives is a sign of poor management.

Hint: The purpose of a computer is to help solve problems.

11. Evaluating Proposals and Vendors

Your RFP is in the hands of the experts now. From the statistical data you provided, the vendor will determine what equipment you currently need and whether or not the system can be upgraded to accommodate your projected growth. Everything will be priced, making it easier for you to make that final decision.

The reliable vendor will thoroughly evaluate your request, breaking it down into many segments, such as ease of operation, instructions, automatic charge tickets, the patient master, accounts receivable, insurance, billing, audit trails, data base, reports, hardware maintenance, technical capabilities, etc. On a point scale, the vendors may rate their system to your requirements. If modifications are necessary, it must be determined whether they are realistically achievable and, if so, at what additional cost.

Let's say that your request include a management report summarizing the services performed at various hospitals. The program for vendor #1 may have been written for the place of service codes and doesn't allow for entry of specific hospitals. It's possible that the modification could not be achieved within a reasonable time frame or that it would be too costly to be considered. The program for vendor #2, however, allows for the hospital names to be entered but does not allow for a summary report. Since the information is in the program, the modification should be easier to achieve at less cost. Vendor #3, on the other hand, may have everything in place and be able to rate your requirement at the highest point on the point scale.

What if you need the report but failed to list it as a requirement in your RFP? All vendors' proposals should be comparatively equal because all systems should provide management reports. What if you have 20 requirements and don't list any in the RFP? Can you see what will happen? The odds are that you won't select the right computer system for your office.

Sales people are sales-oriented, but most won't tell you outright lies. There can be omissions and ambiguities in the way proposals or reports are presented, and this may lead to confusion in the way you interpret these proposals/reports. Sales people are trained to tell you what their product or service will do, not what it won't do.

Providing accurate statistical data will ensure that you get a system that will accommodate your current and future needs, but it does not ensure that the program will work for your practice.

If your RFP is detailed, the vendor should evaluate it step by step with the same scrutiny as used in the example of the report. When the proposal is presented to you, it should be meaningful. It will avoid—or help to avoid—last-minute surprises. You may find that some of your requirements are too costly and cannot be considered or that you're wiling to do some trade-offs. But before you make any decisions, you'll need to evaluate all proposals for determining which systems offer the best solution to your problems within your price range.

Analyze each proposal. Your objective is to select two or three for further evaluation. You'll want to see demonstrations and also visit an office, if possible, that is on the system. You'll check references. You'll constantly be asking questions and taking notes. After all, your primary aim is to select a supplier.

Don't discard the proposals submitted until after you have made your final choice. You may need to go back to the drawing board.

Watch out for programs that allow you to generate your own reports. Remember—if the information you're seeking is not entered into the system, there is no way the computer can generate a report. You may also find that having the capability to design your own reports is so complicated that your staff would not use the function. Insist on seeing this function demonstrated live. Tell the vendor the special report you want generated and watch him/her do it. Don't accept seeing a report that was preprogrammed into this report generator as your guarantee that it can be done. Watch the entire operation.

Select a Supplier

Selecting the right supplier, or vendor, is perhaps the most critical step in shopping for your system. A good vendor will hold your hand through the all-important installation and start-up phase. He'll train you and your office personnel to use the system, show up promptly when your computer goes on the blink, and offer advice when you need it.

But, of course, there are also bad vendors. Some are less than honest. Others are well-meaning, but undercapitalized; they can go bust and leave you high and dry.

So volatile is the computer industry that during a given year many new systems houses—firms that put together entire computer systems for their customers—will spring up, while others go under. A similar success/failure story probably applies to computer retail stores.

THREE BASIC CHOICES. In choosing a vendor, you have three basic choices (not including a service bureau, an option that was discussed in Chapter 4):

- A large, national manufacturer like IBM, NCR Corp., Digital Equipment Corp., or Wang Laboratories Inc.
- A turnkey-systems house—a firm that buys computer components from manufacturers and assembles them into a workable system. It should specialize in medical-office applications.
- A retail store that sells computer components. These computer stores can be independently owned, part of a chain, or backed by a major manufacturer.

No matter which approach you choose, you should subject a potential vendor to a stringent evaluation. Start by checking the firm's financial status.

EVALUATE THE OPERATION. With the big boys, this is relatively easy, since most are traded on the New York or American stock exchange. A call to your broker or a review of the company's listing in Standard & Poor's should suffice. You might also look at the company's most recent annual report.

With smaller vendors, you're on shakier ground, which means you should at least obtain a credit rating from Dun & Bradstreet or other sources. Some retail chains require store owners to have a healthy credit line—$250,000 or more in some cases—thus reducing the risk of financial instability. The manufacturer-owned stores, such as IBM Product Centers, are also secure.

Most consultants say you should shun independent stores, systems houses, and service bureaus that haven't been around for a while. Personally, I won't recommend any company that hasn't been in business for at least three years. I also like it to have a number of installations in medical offices. It should have strong contacts with the company whose computer it sells. It should be a national or at least a large regional firm with strong service and programming departments.

GET REFERENCES. Insist on references. Specify particularly that you want a complete list of the vendor's M.D.-clients. If that means a long list of names, take just those in your specialty. Good vendors will jump at the chance to give you their entire list; problem vendors will try to give you a list of selected names.

Then arrange to visit as many doctors as you have time for, and see their systems in use. Ask questions about the vendor's familiarity with the medical field, problems incurred with contracts or warranties, difficulties during the transition from manual processing to the computer, and get them to recount their computer experience from Day One—both benefits and mistakes.

INTERVIEW THE VENDOR. Prepare an interview outline for seeking additional information that will help you do a comparison analysis of the vendor. The end result is to denote the levels of quantity, quality, or relations so you can rate the vendors by performance standards.

The performance standard analysis should include all measurable facts, such as:

Quantify as much as possible.

- The number of years in business.
- The number of people employed.
  - •• Company officers
  - •• Sales and marketing
  - ••Technical staff (system analysis, programmers, etc.)

(If everyone is in sales and marketing, watch out!)

- The number of systems installed in physicians' offices and in your particular specialty.
- The number of program modules available for a totally integrated system.
- The number of program enhancements to date.(Are they keeping up with the changes affecting medicine?)
- The contractual guarantee for response to downtime.
- The contractual guarantee for on-site response time.
- The number of contracts to be signed for obtaining the system (hardware and software).
- The number of contracts to be signed for maintenance.

Qualify as much as possible. (Rate excellent, good, average, fair, or poor.)

- The company's financial stability.
- Vendor's inventory. (See page 130, Visit the Vendor.)
- Communication skills of the personnel. (See page 130, Visit the Vendor.)

Relation findings.

- The vendor provides a user's manual.
- User group meetings are scheduled periodically.
- The vendor provides a training manual.
- The vendor provides staff training.
  - •• Length of time
  - •• Cost
  - •• Training other employees at a later date (a year or so from now)
- Error and omission insurance (See below).

VISIT THE VENDOR. Visit the firm's office or store. Some of these organizations are so new and poorly financed that you may find the principals working out of their basements. Look for a well-stocked supply room. A substantial inventory of printers, disk drives, and the like is essential if a vendor is to provide good service. Talk to the store manager and the programmers who work with customers. If they speak only computerese or seem too busy to bother with you, take your business elsewhere.

ERROR-AND-OMISSION INSURANCE. Find out whether the prospective vendor carries this insurance. It's a coverage that protects him if you have to sue him because his program ate your practice files. Only the most software-knowledgeable insurers dare sell it (the Chubb Group is one, for example), and only the first rank of vendors qualifies to buy it.

COMPARISON ANALYSIS. After selecting the best proposals and the best vendors, you might find proposal choice #1 comes from vendor choice #8; proposal choice #2, from vendor #5; and, proposal choice #3, from vendor choice #1. But you're ready to make a decision based on information, not assumptions. For example, proposal choice #1 comes from a vendor who has been in business for two years (everything else equal); are you willing to risk that the company will be around to serve your future needs? Suppose proposal #3 will cost you $5,000 more, as compared to choice #1; are you willing to pay the premium dollar to deal with the vendor?

Settle on a System

NARROW THE FIELD. Now you're ready to narrow the field to two or three systems and make a final selection. Here you'll certainly consider cost, but also weigh the terms and conditions of sale, characteristics of the equipment, the vendor's service capability, and so forth.

GET DEMONSTRATIONS. Next, ask for demonstrations of the systems. Block out plenty of time so that you can evaluate each one without being interrupted. Make sure that you see the whole system—the central processing unit, the peripherals (printer, disk drives, terminals, etc.), and the software—in operation. The salesman may show you just the processing unit and tell you that this disk drive or that software program won't be ready for a couple of months. Don't tolerate such tactics. You're buying a machine, not a dream.

RUN A BENCHMARK PROGRAM. Whether you see a system demonstrated in a medical office like yours—the ideal setup—or in the vendor's salesroom, bring along a so-called benchmark program to put the system through its paces. Such a benchmark might consist of a filled-in third-party insurance form, a monthly bill, or a patient-information letter—real-world examples, in other words, of the work you expect the computer to do in your office. Ask the vendor's operators to process this material, and don't accept any alibis if the computer spits out gibberish. If those expert operators can't get good results on such a test, it's unlikely that your untrained assistants will do any better.

HAVE YOUR STAFF TRY IT. It's important to have the people in your office who will be using the system try it out. See if they can understand the accompanying documentation (the instructions on how to operate the computer) and actually operate the system using live data from your practice.

DON'T SHOP FOR PRICE ALONE. Watch out for the supplier who comes in with the lowest bid, especially if it's significantly lower than the others. By taking the lowest bid, you may end up with a system that doesn't have enough storage to handle all your patient records.

Price alone isn't critical, nor is it essential to buy the newest, state-of-the-art computer. What *is* important is to find a computer that will handle your requirements for the long haul. If you buy a computer that will serve your needs for only two years, but you plan to amortize the cost over a five-year period, then you could have a problem.

12. Negotiating the Contract

Negotiate the Deal

Once you've settled on a computer and the financing (see Chapter 9), you'll undoubtedly be impatient to close the deal and get the system running. Don't let your impatience get the better of you. Your future satisfaction may well hinge on the purchase agreement you sign with the vendor. (The assumption is that even if you lease, it will be with a professional leasing company, and that you'll have a separate agreement with your vendor.) Arriving at a proper agreement can take a surprising amount of effort.

STANDARD SALES CONTRACT. No matter which vendor you decide to do business with, you'll probably be given a standard sales agreement to sign. One is pretty much like another, and all are blatantly one-sided: The standard contract overemphasizes the user's responsibility, omits or minimizes the vendor's obligations, and says nothing at all about the vendor's liability for nonperformance.

The first-time computer buyer will usually sign such an agreement without realizing he's playing with a stacked deck—a deck, moreover, that he needn't accept. You have more leverage than you probably realize. Computer companies are hungry for business. They'll usually accommodate you if you're reasonable and know what to ask for.

Examine each position the vendor takes in the contract and ask yourself, "Why?" Their position and your interest will often stimulate the creativity needed for mutually advantageous solutions. Successful negotiation requires being both firm and open.

Success is dependent upon the vendor making a decision you want, and you should do everything possible to help make that decision an easy one. Self-interest is primary, but you also need to place yourself in his shoes. The outcome of the compromise must be fair, legal, and honorable to both parties. The reason you negotiate is to produce something better than the results you obtain without negotiating. What are the alternatives? Protecting yourself against a bad agreement is one thing; producing a good agreement is another.

When negotiating, use questions instead of statements. Statements generate resistance; questions generate answers. You're looking for solutions to the problems, and so is the vendor. Both sides can be winners!

Don't accept a verbal agreement—keep it in writing. For instance, if the system provided does not handle your accounts receivable as outlined in your RFP, negotiate with the vendor that he replace the system with a larger one at no cost to you within a specified time frame. This should keep the vendor from selling you a system that is too small for your needs. Of course, the only way the vendor would probably accept this clause added to the agreement would, no doubt, be contingent upon the accuracy of the information provided by the medical office. Both parties' interest is being protected. And if you thought you were seeing 10 new patients per week and you were actually averaging 20, you provided the vendor with erroneous information, and the clause in the agreement would be null and void if the system proved too small for your needs.

After you have reached a final agreement and everything is in writing, it's usually advantageous to have your attorney look at the contract before signing it. If you have any questions, now is the time to determine the legal implications.

PROTECT YOUR INTERESTS. In order to safeguard your rights and negotiate the best possible deal for yourself, you should follow these ground rules:

Ask for copies of the vendor's contract at the outset of negotiations, so you won't face any surprises later on. And *never* sign the standard contract.

Involve your attorney or professional adviser early enough in the negotiations to allow him to offer suggestions and strengthen your position. And, of course, involve your computer administrator, especially if she's had prior experience in purchasing computer equipment.

Make sure all sales promises are written out. No matter what the salesman promises orally, the courts normally rule that if what he says isn't included in the written contract, it's not legally enforceable. It's a good idea, too, to make your RFP and the vendor's response a part of the contract. The RFP states what the system is supposed to do. The vendor's response amounts to a warranty that the system is fit for a particular purpose.

Delay payment. Most vendors want one-third of their money up front, one-third on delivery, and the balance within 30 days—a schedule that may require you to pay for a system before it's completely debugged. For your protection, don't make the final payment until testing is complete and the system is fully operational. A colleague of mine takes an even harder line. He recommends that you hold back on final payment until two monthly statement-processing routines have been carried out successfully. If the system passes these tests, the vendor gets paid; if not, the vendor keeps working on the system until it passes.

Push for a "drop dead" date. If the vendor is unable or unwilling to meet performance specifications within a time you've both agreed upon, you should be able to walk away from the deal without making the final payment. This date should be set forth in your contract.

Insist that your source code be put in escrow. The source code is the program on which your software is based. Without it, you can't modify or add to your software. If the code is placed in escrow as part of your agreement, you'll always have access to it no matter what happens to the vendor.

Spell out the vendor's liability. The ideal contract should also spell out specific damages for which the vendor is liable if the system doesn't perform properly. Try to get a clause making the vendor liable for your legal fees if you end up in court and win a favorable judgment. You can also place a requirement in the contract for the vendor to provide hardware and software upgrades, when and if they become available, at his expense.

MAKE SURE THE PRICE IS RIGHT. As a final safeguard, ask the vendor to specify in writing that the system has not been sold for less money to anyone else. The vendor is out to get the best deal he can, and it's good business for you, the customer, to do the same. That, after all, is what shopping for a computer system is all about.

13. Should You Pay Cash, Borrow, or Lease?

Once you've determined what your computer system will cost, you have to decide whether you want to purchase it for cash, take out a loan, or simply lease the entire system. And if you're incorporated, you also have to decide *who* will acquire the equipment. But don't make that decision without consulting your CPA and/or tax advisor.

The 1986 Tax Reform Act has resulted in major changes in the taxation of business income, and it still appears that more changes will be forthcoming. This law implemented many new measures to curtail tax shelters, and it also changed the recovery method for depreciable property. The Act also repeals the regular investment tax credit for property placed in service after 1985, except for certain transition property. With all the changes that have occurred, you need your CPA and/or your tax advisor to guide you in making a sound business decision for buying, borrowing, or leasing a computer system. But some general rules do apply.

Financing Arrangements

Now for the more important question of whether to make an outright purchase, take out a loan for purchase, or lease the equipment from a leasing company.

CASH PURCHASE. First of all, remember that it's almost always cheaper to buy than to acquire equipment in any other way (legally, that is). But maybe you don't have $50,000 sitting around—or if you do, you don't want to commit it to a single purchase. Then you have to think about either taking out a loan or leasing the equipment.

BORROWING VERSUS LEASING. Notwithstanding all those fancy four-color brochures from leasing companies, it's almost always less expensive to borrow than to lease. Whenever you do see a work-up by a leasing company, make sure they take it out over a long period of time—say 10 years. Many leasing companies' programs are cheaper in the first years, but you more than make up for this in later years.

How much more expensive is it to borrow than to pay cash? And to lease than to borrow? This will depend on many factors—loan rates, lease rates, prevailing stock-, bond-, and money-market rates, depreciation schedules, and so forth. Leasing will probably prove to be far more expensive than the cash-purchase or loan-for-purchase route.

When It Pays to Lease

YOU CHANGE YOUR MIND. Despite these bottom-line statistics, there are certainly times when it does pay to lease computer equipment. First of all, you only *think* you want a computer system. Many a doctor has run right out and purchased a computer for cash—and now it sits gathering dust because the doctor and his assistants decided they liked the old system better. If you lease and then decide that a computer's not for you, your potential liability will be much less, even if you have to pay penalties to the lessor to get out of a contract.

YOU WANT A NEWER MODEL. Then, you have to remember that the technology of data processing is always changing and improving. The system you purchase today may well do the job for you for many years to come; but a newer system coming out next year may do it more quickly and less expensively. And that new system may even cost less than the one you'll buy today.

YOU'RE CASH-POOR AND CAN'T SWING A LOAN. And, of course, you just might not have either the cash or enough credit to qualify for a loan. If your practice has just purchased expensive clinical equipment, for example, you may find yourself cash-starved. And the banks won't be anxious to advance you more money if you've already got big loans to be paid off.

YOU WANT SPECIAL TERMS. A final feature of leasing is that you can pretty much get the lease structured to your terms. Many leasing companies will work out deals where your first-year costs will be next to nothing—or even nothing—if this fits your budget and your cash flow best. Of course, you'll pay for this service heavily in the later years of the contract, but perhaps you know you'll be better able to afford the payments then.

So you may decide it's a good idea to lease. If you do, here are several points you should consider before you sign a contract.

Contract Considerations

PURCHASE OPTION. Don't lease any computer equipment that you don't have the option of buying at the end of the lease period. At the same time, have a specific purchase figure written into the contract. A number of doctors have been stung because the option was for "fair market value"—as determined by the leasing company. Unscrupulous lessors have placed that value at up to 65 percent of the original cost when a reasonable figure might have been 25 percent or less.

OBSOLESCENCE PROTECTION. This should be an item that you negotiate hard on, especially if a big reason for leasing is that you're afraid new technology might make your system obsolete. Try to insert a clause in the contract that will allow you to cancel the lease if a newer version of the same equipment makes your model obsolete. *If* you can get such a contract, you should also have the option to negotiate a new lease for the newer model.

HIDDEN COSTS. Many equipment-leasing plans make the lessee fully responsible for maintenance, repairs, and casualty losses. Find out what you're responsible for. If fire destroys your computer system and your insurance doesn't cover the loss, you may end up paying for it out of your own pocket. The contract should spell out who pays personal property taxes, if any, on the equipment.

If you follow these tips, you should end up with a lease you can live with. But as noted earlier, your first choice should still be the cash-purchase route, followed closely by the loan for purchase.

The cost of the loan is dependent upon the annual rate of interest. A $50,000 loan at 12 percent interest financed for 60 months will cost $66,733.20. If, however, you could negotiate the same loan and terms at a 10 percent annual interest rate, the cost would decrease to $63,741.00, a savings of $2,992.20.

As emphasized in the beginning, before you make a decision and certainly before you sign any papers, meet with your CPA and/or tax advisor. Their expertise may save you from making a costly mistake and should help ensure that you receive the greatest return on your investment.

14. Before Your Computer Arrives

Planning Checklist

In planning for the arrival of your new computer, nothing is as important as the plan itself—a checklist of things to be done and their target dates for completion. Items on the list should include preparing and training employees, getting your site ready for the new equipment, insuring your investment, converting your present system to the electronic one, notifying your patients, and so forth.

You'll have to brace yourself for a possibly stormy transition period. Your staff's learning to live with a computer system demands a great deal of leadership on your part. There are practical and emotional considerations to deal with. There are a lot of dynamics to the process, and the atmosphere in your office will change dramatically.

That means that you must be personally involved in all the aspects of your office that will be affected by the computer. How involved? Enough to know, in broad outline, how the system operates and what the changes will be. You don't need hands-on knowledge. But neither should you be alien to the computer system, subservient to it, or intimidated by it. The game plan should be *yours,* and you should be the one who monitors its progress.

The basic items on your checklist are these:

1. Staff preparation—assigning roles and responsibilities; appointing someone to plan the activities, allocate the responsibilities, and evaluate progress
2. Training—arranging for formal meetings, orientation, and other involvement
3. Site preparation—making whatever architectural, electrical, and mechanical arrangements are necessary, as well as redesigning or rearranging desks, cabinets, and other furniture
4. Supplies—ordering the forms and various accessories that must be in the office before the new equipment can be operated
5. Conversion—handling all the details necessary to guarantee that the process of converting from your manual system to the new electronic one will be as easy and problem-free as possible.

Preparing Your Staff

The sooner employees get involved in the installation, the better. Presumably, you've already involved them during the decision-making process (as discussed in Chapter 5). They should even have participated somewhat in the shopping. But your selling job hasn't ended. As arrival day nears, you should still be boosting the good system and the easier life your staff is about to encounter, getting them talking positively about what they'll be able to do with the new system and how much it will do for them.

HOLD PERIODIC MEETINGS. Meetings should be held periodically with your staff. They should be well planned—format, procedure, sequence, objectives. Assuming you've kept your personnel well informed and have used their input to select your system, the teamwork process has gradually been developing. Since changing office technology creates higher job stress as well as new and often greater responsibilities, these meetings must be designed to prepare the staff for all the objectives to be accomplished.

The positive mental attitudes you're helping to build will go a great way toward alleviating the fear of change and reducing the stress factor. Properly preparing the staff should help improve their ability to deal with problems—both people problems and situation problems. It should also help them make the most of their new job opportunities, which will in turn increase the effectiveness of the office.

EMPHASIZE TEAMWORK. One person cannot do the job successfully; it requires teamwork. Changes in procedures cannot simply be announced; they must be planned, prepared for. Your staff will be more organized and will communicate more effectively as a direct result of this planning and preparation.

POST ASSIGNMENTS. An assignment chart must be developed to include each task, the person responsible for it, the target date for completion, and a space to record the actual date of completion. There will be times when one task must be completed before another one can begin. It's imperative to know whether assignments are being completed as scheduled, or whether people are sitting around waiting for others.

It will cost you dearly if the computer arrives before all the tasks have been completed. A system sitting around unused is sucking money from your pocket. And trying to implement the system without being fully prepared only serves to increase the chance of failure.

ENCOURAGE YOUR STAFF. Even with all this preparation, you'll still face some initial resistance, especially among the veteran employees. You may suffer some staff turnover. Many a doctor has even abandoned his computer plans when faced with the defection of valued staff members. Try to hang in there. If applicable, remind your people how they resisted modernizing attempts in the past—a move to new quarters, for example, or electric typewriters, third-party billing procedures, new clinical equipment, and the like. Remind them that this is *their* system, not yours. *They're* the ones who'll benefit the most.

If you can, discover other medical or dental offices in your area that have successfully computerized, and arrange discussions between their employees and yours. (A little screening on your part is called for. First make sure that your people won't be subjected to a litany of horror stories about early problems, mistakes, and failures, or the story of poor old Margaret, who quit after 35 years of valued service because she just couldn't cope with the newfangled gadgetry.)

BE PATIENT. No matter how much you try to convince your employees that the new system and its benefits are *theirs,* the fact remains that the impetus and enthusiasm for it are largely yours. So don't push them too fast. Don't set unrealistically short target dates for getting the system on line. Consider modifying your office schedule to allow ample learning time, and to allow reluctant employees to get used to the idea of computerization. Emphasize praise, motivation, and confidence-building pep talks.

This patience on your part should be viewed as more than just an emotional consideration—it's a practical one as well. The fact is, any medical assistant will have trouble learning the computer *and* handling the normal patient flow at the same time. At the least, you may have to reduce your staff's workload or give them time periods during the day just to get acquainted with the system. You may even find it worthwhile to hire part-time or temporary help so your regular employees will have time for learning.

Training

FORMAL SESSIONS WITH THE VENDOR. There should be formal instructional sessions available from the vendor for several employees in your office. These sessions should be held away from the office, if possible. The staff will have more time to digest, absorb, and play with what they've learned. Those who'll work with the computer most closely should be able to train other employees. Try to have at least one backup employee who can fill in when each regular operator is out. Otherwise you'll have to revert to manual operation.

The amount of training your staff is entitled to depends on your contract with the vendor. Negotiate for as much as possible. Figure at least three to five full days of training. But be aware that you will have to pay for additional or future training, so make sure you get all you need as part of your basic contract. Otherwise, you'll be like so many doctors who can't get their $50,000 systems fully operational

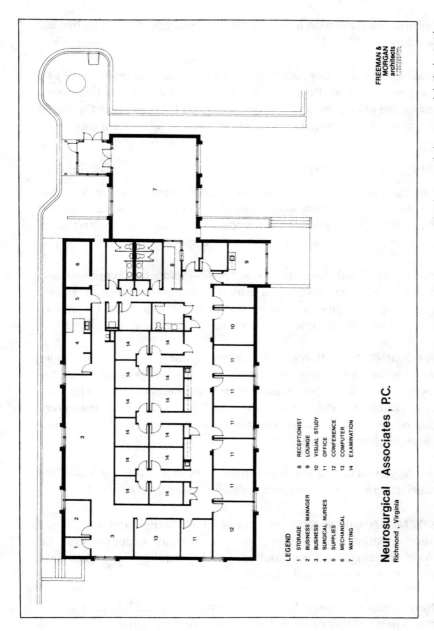

Figure 14-1. *Office layout for a six-doctor, computerized specialty practice. The layout of the room labeled 13 (the computer room) is shown in more detail in Fig. 14-2.*

because they and their assistants received inadequate training by their vendors.

How long before your people are ready to fly on their own? There's no pat answer to that. Partly, it depends on each employee. If someone grasps the principles quickly, she may be ready before the trainer's out the door. If an employee struggles, she may struggle for a year.

Site Preparation

You can't just jam your computer into a congested corner or inaccessible extra room. Unfortunately, though, most medical offices were not planned with an in-house data-processing system in mind, and space tends to be at a premium. So what do you do?

You prepare, with the emphasis on "pre"—*before* the computer is due to arrive. You may want to do extensive architectural, electrical, and mechanical rearranging. Or you may need only to move a couple of file cabinets. But in any case, you must anticipate all your needs.

PLACEMENT OF HARDWARE. It is often desirable to locate the printer and one terminal close to where the action is, generally near the receptionist's desk (though away from patient traffic). The central processing unit, or CPU, can go down the hall or in the extra bathroom. But no two practices are exactly alike. Analyze your own needs closely before you decide.

A diagram showing the placement of the hardware, including the work stations for the terminals, should be drawn (see Fig. 14-2).

SPECIAL REQUIREMENTS. Ask your vendor whether your system will need anything in particular in order to function properly—special floor covering, heating, cooling, wiring, lighting, soundproofing, ventilation, or structural support.

New wiring is the most likely accommodation you'll have to make. You'll need antisurge devices to protect your system from electrical fluctuations, and possibly an antistatic mat (though most new ma-

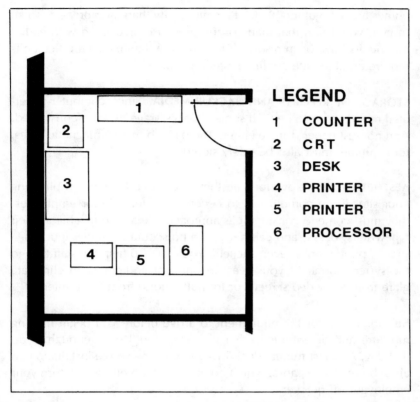

Figure 14-2. *Model layout sketch of a typical data-processing center in a medical office.*

chines are less vulnerable to static electricity than their predecessors). In fact, you'll find that many of the problems associated with earlier computers have been resolved; for example, few medical-office units require an elaborate cooling system anymore.

STORAGE OF REPORTS AND BACKUP MEDIA. Since computer-generated reports have to be filed somewhere, storage must be considered. And not just paper storage either. The backup media (magnetic tapes, for example) must also be safely stored.

AESTHETICS. Don't overlook aesthetic considerations when planning your site. If the computer is to become comfortable for employees, they must come to consider it as approachable and touchable as their typewriters, desks, and cabinets. Don't discourage homey touches— plants, photographs, even stickers. You can also help the staff take to the system sooner if you invest in optional equipment to eliminate glare from the video screens or to muffle noise from the printer.

But don't wait for the equipment to arrive before you begin moving furniture and determining other changes. You'll have enough to do that day. And last-minute decisions will give the whole installation an air of hysteria and panic, which nobody needs. Nothing will turn your employees off quicker.

ASSIGNING THE JOB. Site preparation is an assigned task that should be well planned, with a target date set for completion. If there are special preparation requirements, a checklist should be used. This is generally a job for your computer administrator.

Supplies

Even with the best of systems, nothing will happen if you don't have the forms, reports, tapes, ribbons, bills, and paper you need. All of it should be ordered well in advance and received prior to the arrival of the equipment. Your computer administrator should be able to work with the vendor's salesman in ordering the necessary items. Don't overlook even the smallest of details:

- It may be necessary to design or redesign the statement used for billing.
- In your design of statement envelopes, be sure to include any applicable postal information such as "presorted mail" or "forwarding address requested."
- Source documents (such as the charge slip, or fee slip) should be designed for ease of computer entry, so the operator won't have to scan an entire sheet of records for the required information.
- Forms should be continuous and perforated for easy separation. They should also contain all the necessary information for third-party billing. (The continuous universal insurance claim form can be purchased from the AMA; Blue Cross-Blue Shield will provide the continuous forms for submitting their claims.)

Insurance and Security

HARDWARE AND SOFTWARE COVERAGE. Don't overlook insurance protection. Your agent can help you decide whether you should have a rider on your current office insurance policy or a separate policy for the computer system. Your coverage can be either minimal or elaborate—from bare-bones fire-and-theft coverage of hardware only, to protection against the loss of valuable tapes and disks. But the best—and safest—idea is probably to cover the replacement cost of all hardware and software. You might also wish to insure against losses due to computer downtime.

FIRE PROTECTION. Computer hardware is susceptible to fire damage. Industry experts now agree that only one type of fire extinguisher—the Halon (halogenated hydrogen) type—should be recommended for fires involving electronic data-processing equipment. Other kinds of fire extinguishers can damage the hardware as much as a fire.

Halon fire extinguishers should be checked periodically for decreased gas pressure; the gas is colorless and odorless and can ooze away undetected. A Halon fire extinguisher should be mounted in your data-processing area along with smoke and heat detectors. Such equipment may reduce your insurance premiums.

EMBEZZLEMENT PROTECTION. One thing insurance won't protect you against is embezzlement. The threat is small as long as employees aren't familiar enough with the computer to play games with it. That won't, of course, last forever. It may not be long before a clever operator can alter numbers up or down with no physical evidence of any tampering.

One safeguard is to limit computer employees to specified functions and files only, rather than allowing each access to the entire system (see Chapter 7). That keeps any one employee from becoming so familiar with the machine that she's tempted to go into business for herself. But you might feel that it is more important for all your staff members to be familiar with the entire system and to be able to backstop one another with no significant loss of efficiency. You must decide for yourself how you wish to handle this trade-off.

If you feel you might be a mark, set up methods of cross-checking figures. Try batching the daysheets, then running control tapes for a certain period, and comparing the tapes with the totals on the computer and those totals with the computer's regular reports.

Heading off embezzlement can be one function of the computer administrator. If there's a discrepancy, he or she should be responsible for tracking it down.

Conversion From a Manual to a Computerized System

The transition from a manual system to a computer will go smoothly only if your manual system is working smoothly to begin with. If your office is running on a hit-or-miss basis, the computer could actually be destructive.

Don't be misled by the doctor who claims his new computer system has found $20,000 in unknown accounts receivable. If he was losing as much as $20,000 a year without a computer, he could lose twice that much with one.

Preparation of Codes

Various types of coding must be established during the planning or preconversion period. The time when you're actually converting is no time to start gathering data, determining codes, or abbreviating information. If all decisions are made and worksheets completed prior to the actual conversion, a smooth transition is closer to becoming a reality.

Standard industry codes have been established so that doctors can communicate in a uniform language. The Current Procedural Terminology (CPT) code designates medical, surgical, and diagnostic services. It's administered by the AMA, and is available in book form as well as on magnetic computer tapes for easy entry into a data-processing system. The International Classification of Diseases (ICD) is a coded system for diagnoses, symptoms, complaints, and/or reasons for seeking medical attention. The specialized coding needs for any practice can be extracted from either of these sources.

Uniformity of coding is important, because several digits can reveal a lot of information about a patient's medical condition. Consequently, the accuracy of coding cannot be overemphasized. Reliable data are essential. Accurate codes must be maintained for every patient.

During the preconversion period, write down the most common diagnoses and procedures handled in your practice—use separate lists for diagnoses and procedures. The computer system should allow the operator to add or delete diagnoses or procedures whenever needed, but it's important to begin the automation process with those that are common to your specialty or practice. (Some systems may have the diagnosis file already established.)

When establishing coding systems, try to keep in mind what your objectives will be. For example, if you want to know the amount of money collected from various primary insurance companies, establish a code for each insurer—and post payments according to the applicable code.

Input-Options Worksheets

To build the computer files for your practice, you must record all the information on input-options worksheets for the computer operator.

PROCEDURE AND DIAGNOSIS FILES. Your codes must be acceptable to third-party payers. There are also a limited number of character spaces allowed for describing each procedure or diagnosis; you can't exceed that limit. Abbreviations may become necessary. How would you abbreviate "laminectomy for decompression of spinal cord and/or cauda equina, more than two segments; cervical" to fit in 40 character spaces? You also need to price the procedures. If you have several fee schedules, worksheets must be prepared for each one.

CODING CODES. Some software packages even allow for the *coding of codes*. For example, "9" may represent CPT procedure code 63015 (the laminectomy above). So if the computer operator entered "9," the system would automatically enter the procedure as 63015—but only one keystroke would be required instead of five. Shortening the keypunch operation speeds up the entire process.

INSURANCE CODES. You might want to assign separate codes to Blue Shield, Medicare, workers' compensation, CHAMPUS, and "other commercial insurance carriers." Or you might want to assign a separate code to each primary commercial carrier, such as Aetna, Hartford, Metropolitan, Travelers, and the rest.

Financial classifications of accounts must be determined and coded so the system knows which type of insurance form to generate and which detailed data to provide on which form. Each account can be assigned a financial classification, with the code perhaps a single number or one or two letters. A Blue Shield financial classification account, for example, could carry the code "1" or "BS," depending on how the program is written.

OTHER PAYER CODES. Then you'd want to assign codes to other categories for which you'd want to track payments—cash, personal check, money order, welfare payments, payments by attorneys, and any other specific source that generated income for the practice. If any category listed and coded as a payment center actually withdraws money on a payment voucher to correct a payment error, it's necessary to have specific payment centers for the withdrawal accounts.

ACCOUNT-ADJUSTMENT CODES. Adjustments to patient accounts would include general classes such as bad debts, reductions, professional courtesy, bankruptcy, refunds, check returned from the bank for various reasons, and charity. It's also essential to set up the kinds of adjustment codes best suited to the needs of your practice, which will provide the detailed information *you* feel is important to know. If, for example, you accept Medicare assignments and want to know the dollar amount you write off each month—the difference between your charge and the allowable charge determined by the insurer—a special code can be set up for this adjustment. The more detailed you are, the better the information will be. Make your computer work for you.

Special handling of accounts requires a separate coding system. If you want to accept insurance as payment in full on an account, you should have the ability to program it into the computer. You wouldn't want that patient to be billed for services rendered, or to be sent a follow-up bill even though the account has been paid by a third party.

If the system allows for special handling of accounts, will the insurance claim forms be computer generated, or must they be done by hand? Any account that requires special handling should be able to be incorporated into the system. If any manual work is required for special handling, it should be documented, with a staff member assigned to complete the job.

REVENUE-CENTER CODES. Codes may also be necessary for revenue centers. Most practices find it helpful, for example, to know just how much income is generated from which source—from surgery, lab testing, injections, diagnostic procedures, hospital patients, office patients, consultations, etc. This coding should also be tailored to meet your specific needs.

PHYSICIAN CODES. Each physician in your practice will be assigned a code, and a record kept of each service the doctor performs. In addition, if there are multiple office locations, each office site should be coded. Place-of-service codes (e.g., hospital, office) are usually established according to the recognized universal codes as listed on the insurance forms.

For printing out information as hard copy, the computer can be programmed to convert the codes into the information they actually represent: "17" can be printed out as "Dr. Jones"; "1" as "Blue Shield"; "44" as "tonsillectomy." Some statements and forms, however, may not have space for the printed-out version; these the computer would have to print in code. Therefore, take into consideration when the statement is designed how much information you want to appear on the form. It's taking care of details such as this that paves the way for a smooth conversion.

OPTIONS TO SUIT YOUR NEEDS. Options available on an adaptable prepackaged software program can allow you to design some features to suit your particular needs. It's important, for example, to determine how many spaces are available for designating payment and adjustment codes. Some programs restrict you to 10 or 12 codes, while others permit 100. If you need 25 payment codes and the system allows for only 15, you have a problem. (Presumably, this would have been a consideration during the selection process.)

Assigning Account Numbers

Assigning account numbers to patients' accounts takes planning. You must know, for example, how many character or digit spaces the system allows for an account number. If the program allows for only eight, you can't assign accounts by nine-digit Social Security numbers. If your practice already has an account-numbering system, can the computer program accommodate it? Some programs allow only for digits in account numbers, whereas others allow for letters as well.

Other questions to ask: Does the account number provide you with any basic information, or is it just a numbering system? Is the account-numbering system planned so that it guarantees you won't run out of numbers? Does the system generate and assign account numbers that can be used for your practice?

If your practice has never used account numbers, the system will have to be determined from scratch. In addition, all the account numbers must be recorded on the patients' medical charts manually—and that includes a massive checking and rechecking job to make sure no errors are made.

Does the system allow for collection letters? If so, those letters must be composed for accounts according to an aging analysis. A message for an account that is 30 days old, for example, would have a much different tone ("please," or "prompt payment appreciated") from messages that go out for three-month-old unpaid bills. Your computer program may limit messages to a maximum number of characters and spaces. Composing messages within those limitations requires planning, and you'll probably write several drafts before you have exactly what you want.

Other decisions to be made: Do you want to continue to send bills for accounts with balances that have fallen below some minimum amount? Do you want to send statements for credit balances? Do you want to send zero-balance statements? Most doctors say No.

Do you want to use *patient* billing (in which each individual patient has an account) or *family* billing (in which all members of a family are put on one account)? This decision should also be made during the preconversion period. The information needed for input into the computer for either type of billing system, as well as methods for obtaining that information, should be discussed at this time. Source documents should be ready so that the operator can start keying directly into the computer, without having to hunt around for data or wait for last-minute decisions, once the computer system is in place.

You may want to notify your patients, and certainly some of your more prominent third-party payers, that you're converting to a computer.

Your patients should become more willing to accept a balance forward on their accounts (though a method of billing should be worked out to assure their receiving itemized bills for any current services prior to the computerized statement).

Third-Party-Payer Requirements

You should work out with your third-party providers any considerations attached to the conversion. Will computerizing affect the promptness of payment on claims? Will there be any problems with the exchange of information? Does the insurer need more, or less, detailed information to process its claims?

Since certain requirements must be met before the insurer can honor claims, a trial run of some computer-generated claims may be indicated. Your third-party payers can also provide you with invaluable input. They deal with all manner of computerized claims and can steer you away from potentially rocky waters.

PATIENTS' SIGNATURES ON FILE. For example, patients' signatures must appear on all insurance claim forms for processing. If the benefits are to be paid directly to the physician, a second patient signature is required. Most insurance companies will accept a photocopy of these authorizations from a standard form completed by the patient for the medical office. The words "signature on file" can be programmed into the computer system for printing in the blocks designed for a signed authorization. But some insurers require that a copy of the patient's signed authorization be attached to the computer-generated claim before it's submitted. Working this out with your insurers beforehand should help you avoid delays in processing and receiving payments.

Medicare, for one, has special requirements regarding "signature on file." All Medicare's requirements must be met whether or not you accept assignment, and an audit of the signatures on file can be performed at any time. It would be wise to review Medicare requirements prior to any decision regarding the best method for implementing computer-generated claim processing for your office.

HOOK UP TO AN INSURANCE COMPANY'S COMPUTER. It's sometimes possible to submit insurance claims directly from your computer to the insurer's computer via telephone lines or tapes, but the computers must be compatible. If you have a large volume of claims to be filed with one carrier in particular—Blue Shield, Medicare, or a commercial carrier—that carrier can provide you the information you'll need to investigate or implement "paperless" claim processing. You'll also need to do some test runs.

WHAT IF YOU DON'T PROCESS CLAIMS? Some medical offices do not complete insurance claims for patients and will only provide the essential information on an itemized statement (a "multipurpose billing form"), which the patient can attach to his claim form (see Chapter 17). But even here, with the patient responsible for payment of services rendered, a computer system can aid and enhance personal services provided to and for patients.

Input of Outstanding Accounts

Your accounts receivable—*not* your master patient file—must be put into the computer system as quickly as possible. There must be planning here, too. Only the active accounts should be put on the computer at first. Putting zero-balance accounts on is a waste of time; they can be added if and when these patients return for medical care.

If you're converting from a totally manual system, you must decide how input will be accomplished and whether it will be done by staff or an outside source. If staffers do it, they'll become familiar with the computer more quickly, but may take longer to get the job done. It generally requires the participation of different people and more than one conversion cycle. If an outside source does this job, it will get done faster, but a good deal more expensively. And if it's done outside, your staff may first have to prepare the documents for input into the computer.

To convert your accounts receivable file from a service bureau or other computer system, tape is generally the best medium. This information should have been gathered, prior to selecting your new in-house system. If your files must go to hard copy, you'll encounter essentially the same process as converting from a manual system.

III. Making Your Computer Do Everything You Want It To

15. Once Your Computer's in Place

It's here!

Assuming that adequate space for the equipment has been properly planned and all electrical requirements have been met, installation of the equipment itself should be comparatively simple. The hardware can be placed in the desired location according to plan (Chapter 14), and the peripherals of the system wired from their physical locations to the CPU.

Last-Minute Adjustments

The vendor's field engineer will probably need to do some diagnostic work on the system to assure that everything is in working order, and the vendor's systems analyst will probably need to check the applications and operating-system software, doing any necessary work for implementing and running the system. Your system will then be ready for use and for the building of files. But many last-minute "big day" adjustments remain.

SECURITY FILE. The system should provide for security. By building the security file (an actual computer file stored on the disk), the computer administrator should be able to control the functions the computer operators can perform. The operators should be given assigned passwords that will allow access to the system. If there are three terminals, for example, each operator might be restricted (by security restrictions associated with their passwords in the security file) to one terminal and/or one function to perform (such as account inquiry). One operator could only *look* at patients' accounts or obtain hard copies of them (read-only access) but be unable to put any information into the system (edit access). Or one operator might have access to all the terminals and be allowed to perform several functions, such as posting charges and handling file maintenance.

PASSWORD. Are there any rules about selecting a password? As a matter of fact, there are. Each operator should be assigned a *unique* (and confidential) password for security purposes. You might even change the passwords quarterly—certainly whenever an operator terminates employment. Operators should *never* reveal their passwords to others, and should not keep them written down in an accessible place. Passwords are designed for operators' protection, and for the security of the system. Choose passwords that cannot easily be guessed—avoid using first names, initials, or other obvious codes.

VIDEO-SCREEN AND HARD-COPY OUTPUT. It is wishful thinking to believe that a breach of security could not occur in a small medical office or on a small computer system. Even simple carelessness can cause breaches of security. A terminal located where unauthorized persons can view the video screen could be a serious security breach. Hard-copy output must be destroyed or filed, not just thrown into a wastebasket where anyone can read it. These security measures are necessary to guarantee patients' privacy.

Building Computer Files

If you completed the input-options worksheets during the preconversion period (Chapter 14), you should be ready to build the files into the computer. From the worksheets, the computer administrator or operator can build right into the system the diagnosis records, the procedure and service fee records, all other option records, and all the necessary information to customize the system to your specific medical practice. Such things as physicians' names and ID numbers (for Medicare and Medicaid, and the DEA authority, for example) and the name and address of the practice will now all be programmed into your system.

The conversion of accounts receivable—again, *not* your master file—will take time. All the information on these accounts must be put into the memory. The computer may be able to store more information than what's on your ledger cards; omitting any basic information is almost sure to decrease efficiency.

PATIENT VERSUS FAMILY BILLING. The choice between the two forms of billing—patient billing and family billing—should have been made during the preconversion period (Chapter 14). Preparations should already have been made enabling the operator to easily key account information into the system from source documents.

IN-HOUSE VERSUS OUTSIDE KEYBOARDING. As mentioned in Chapter 14, keying all your accounts receivable into the computer is tedious and time-consuming. By now you should have decided who will do it: an outside source or your staff. In weighing the advantages and disadvantages of each, keep one overriding goal in mind: accuracy.

AUDITING BALANCES FORWARDED. After all the accounts receivable are put into the computer, a transaction is posted to each account showing a balance forward. There should be financial controls for auditing the total balances forwarded, and also a printed transaction journal showing each account that had recorded activity. The operator should be able to post, for example, 100 or more accounts and then check for accuracy. If she can do this, she'll easily catch and correct discrepancies. When an entry has been posted incorrectly, it usually becomes necessary to back out the entire entry and then post it all over again, correctly this time. Auditing is an essential function, and the computer administrator must know the system and how to audit it.

Parallel Processing
Versus Immediate Conversion

There are two general approaches to conversion once the files have been built: parallel processing, where you operate manually and on the computer simultaneously for a while, and immediate conversion with no manual backup. Which is better? Each has its advantages and disadvantages.

PARALLEL PROCESSING

Disadvantages. Parallel processing, or parallel running, in which you maintain dual systems, is often difficult and requires more-than-double effort, since the new system is operated side by side with the old one until the new system is proved to be operating correctly. Furthermore, the output of both systems must be compared. When discrepancies are found, your staff may need a great deal of time to analyze the results and solve the problems. Sometimes, if the two systems are radically different, comparisons are virtually impossible.

Advantages. Why do it, then? The main advantage to parallel processing is that bugs—errors in program, data, or hardware function—are usually detected early and can be corrected without much downtime. An interesting sidelight: The discrepancies that are found during parallel processing are usually traced to errors in the *manual* system.

Also, parallel processing affords a readily available backup medium that can be used as a standard for testing and evaluating computer processing. And if there are any bugs in the computer program, you've kept the old system up to date so you can fall back on it.

Duration. Parallel processing should not last longer than a few months. As soon as the computer system is proved to be operating correctly, the old system should be discontinued. It's unfair to your staff to wait.

Personnel problems. Duties must be well defined for parallel processing to succeed. Since it's a stressful period because of the extra volume of work, you must be understanding and observant. People under stress often attempt to handle more work than they can accomplish. Once you and your staff are over this hurdle, though, computer processing should begin to enhance your business office efficiency.

IMMEDIATE CONVERSION. The immediate conversion method is commonly known as the "guts" method. The old system stops one day and the new system begins the next. There's no system to fall back on when bugs are found, and your staff may have to reconstruct your old system manually if the new one does not perform satisfactorily. It indeed takes guts to use this method, but if everything goes well it can be to your advantage. It's also much easier on your assistants.

Before going live with the new system, you must compare the output of both systems and resolve any discrepancies. The total for your accounts receivable must be the same on both systems, or so close to the same that you're comfortable with the results.

Some people recommend the guts method of conversion; I don't.

Automated Conversion

To change or upgrade from any form of electronic data-processing system to another is usually easier than from a manual system—unless the information must be put into hard copy before the conversion can occur. If that's the case, it becomes basically the same operation as converting from a manual system. The change, however, is usually not as traumatic for your staff since they're already somewhat familiar with electronic data processing—not a small point to consider.

But it's also essential in this kind of conversion to be just as thorough and complete with your evaluation and planning as if you were converting from manual. Shortcuts can be detrimental to the process. You must know what you have, what you're getting, and all the effects—good and bad—it will have on your practice. Corrective measures can be planned or solutions found for any foreseeable problems.

PRELIMINARY WORK. While automated conversion of accounts receivable transfers the data electronically, all the preliminary work should be done before the arrival of the computer. Once the computer is in house, your efforts should be directed toward getting it into operation as quickly as possible.

PATIENT STATEMENTS. With automated conversion of accounts receivable, the balances forward of the amounts due on patients' accounts are simply transferred to the new system. In fairness to your patients, they should receive statements for their current transactions under the old system before you implement the new one.

SOURCE DOCUMENTS. The accounts receivable data for billing and collection purposes should also be electronically transferable, but the source documents may have to be revised if the advanced program can store more information than the old system could, as is probably the case.

ADDING TO THE FILES. When converting manually, you would put in only the current accounts receivable. But when you're converting electronically, you may also have the capability to transfer your entire master file of zero-balance accounts to the new system. Resist this temptation! It can only load up the new system with information on patients who may never return.

It's usually more efficient to print out and store hard copy on zero-balance accounts. When a patient does return, your assistant can retrieve the hard copy and enter the information into the system and/or have the patient complete an updated registration form. New-patient information, of course, is input either directly during the interview or from (revised) source documents.

KEYBOARDING NEEDS. Although automated conversion of patient records is likely to be much quicker and easier than conversion from a manual system, not all the data in the old computer may be electronically transferable. Plan with your computer administrator for at least a modicum of keyboard work—maybe more.

AUDITS. Audits are essential. The financial data must be the same on both systems. Audits can be accomplished by comparing computer-generated financial reports. Both systems must show the same total number of accounts. Also, run spot checks of informational data on both systems, and obtain hard copies of important reports, including the accounts receivable.

Printing out the accounts receivable could be the very last thing you do on the old system and the first thing you do before actually implementing the new system. The comparative data could be invaluable if any problems arise under the new system.

Running Your Practice While You Convert

The major problem during conversion is that the practice must continue. Patients won't stop getting sick just because you're putting in a computer system. So it is vital for your planning to include maintenance of the normal daily functions of the business while you're still completing the conversion process. For example, as mentioned in Chapter 14, it is often a good idea to hire part-time or temporary help to allow your staff more time to learn the new system.

After all the tasks have been completed, you're ready to run live with your new computer system. You've advanced from having a tested system to having an operational one. Now the actual changeover from the old system to the new one should be simple. You and your computer administrator have done everything possible to ensure a smooth transition. But, with all your planning and preparation, there will be errors—errors from the old system that have been transferred to the new one, as well as some brand-new discrepancies.

Don't worry. Before long, you'll be running at maximum efficiency and the computer will seem as comfortable to everyone as a well-broken-in shoe. Will problems continue to occur? Naturally, just as with any other system—manual or electronic—you've used. Will you be able to handle them just as easily? You bet.

16. Management and Control of Your Date-Processing Procedures

After you've entered your accounts receivable, you'll have to process all your codes and data into your new computer data base. Your computer will probably be programmed to provide a "menu," or list of available tasks (see Fig. 7-1), for the selection of work to be performed and, in addition, lead-through messages or questions to assist the operator in accomplishing her duties.

The Importance of Multiprogramming

Multiprogramming refers to a computer system's ability to handle a number of programs concurrently (and apparently simultaneously) by interleaving their execution. It is actually a type of time sharing of machine components. Most computer systems these days do have some form of multiprogramming.

PROBLEMS IF YOU DON'T HAVE IT. In any medical office, time must be allocated for the staff to look up accounts when patients call with questions. Even in a small practice, this is likely to occur several times a day. If your system has no multiprogramming capability (and there are still some systems lacking it), it may be necessary to tell these patients that the information will be obtained later in the day and someone will get back to them. (Switching back and forth among tasks is often very inefficient in a non-multiprogrammed system. Stopping prior to completion of a task may require starting it again from the beginning.) Since you're so restricted with such a system, the day's activities must be especially well planned, and management of processing time is of primary importance.

HOW TO USE IT EFFECTIVELY. Multiprogramming, on the other hand, allows for several functions to be performed at once. One terminal could be used mainly for account inquiry while other work is being performed at other terminals. If there are three terminals, one operator could be doing patient registration, one could be posting transactions, and the third could be available for inquiry.

To utilize any system fully, of course, work must still be well planned. Some systems allow for all transactions, charges, payments, and adjustments to be posted in the same file, while others may require charges to be posted in one file and payments and adjustments in another. If all transactions are posted in the same file, demand statements can be obtained faster. The time lag due to moving in and out of files, although individually small, still slows down the efficiency of overall performance.

PLANNING PRINTER TIME. If there are several terminals but only one printer, and if you need to do demand statements—statements that patients request—it's necessary to set aside specially designated hours for demand statements to be printed, and use the rest of the time to print transaction journals, reports, insurance forms, regular statements, and the rest.

Constantly moving different kinds of paper and forms in and out of a printer reduces efficiency. You may just find that you need two printers to be able to provide demand statements while getting the regular paperwork accomplished (see Fig. 8-1).

Developing Controls

Entering data into the computer is the easy part. Developing controls for the system to ensure maximum benefits from it takes thoughtful planning.

CONTROLS FOR POSTING CHARGE TRANSACTIONS. It takes only seconds to post a charge transaction and update a patient's account. The patient's account number or name is entered into the system, and the account appears on the video screen. The operator usually verifies that it's the correct account, and then enters the procedure, diagnosis, physician, location codes, and the date(s) the services were rendered. The account has now been updated. That's it! It's a simple procedure, and the next transaction can now be posted. But developing the controls for posting charge transactions is not that simple—it's an ongoing process requiring periodic review and evaluation.

Processing the data for a charge transaction to be entered into the computer system is also relatively easy, but the interrelated work required to reach the processing stage and then maintain control of the necessary functions to help ensure a successful operation is complex.

If you have a sophisticated system that allows for entry of more detailed information, such as dates of disability, return appointment date, authorization numbers, drugs prescribed, etc., the additional data may be recorded on the charge slip and entered into the system when charges are posted. Controls need to be established for auditing the accuracy of the data, and can be accomplished by using the input worksheets to randomly check the entered information.

CHARGE SLIP DESIGN. Initially, a charge slip, or fee slip, must be designed. It may even be necessary to design two—one to accommodate the charges for services rendered to office patients, and the other for hospitalized patients (particularly if surgery is being performed). It also must be designed to allow for ease of keypunching the information into the system. The charge slip must be completed with accurate information; an incorrect diagnosis or procedure could create major insurance and other problems. (Many systems will generate a prenumbered charge slip.)

AVERTING GIGO. Without proper planning and management, control of the system can be virtually impossible and data processing can make one big permanent mess of your business operations. The primary reasons for failure of a computer system are usually lack of planning, management, and/or control.

The acronym GIGO—garbage in, garbage out—didn't appear out of a blue sky. But GIGO operations will inevitably compound the costs of your investment and guarantee the failure of your system. Electronic data processing can enhance your efficiency and business operations only if you're willing to accept the fact that management and control of the system are *not built into the computer* but must come from the resources found within your office.

THE COMPUTER ADMINISTRATOR'S ROLE. Once your office is on the new computer system, the computer administrator should not only audit the work performed but also constantly review and evaluate the overall performance of both the system and the personnel involved. Good accounting procedures should always be maintained. Don't be afraid to revise or change the existing plan to achieve better performance or control.

Control of Patient Data

NEW PATIENTS. New-patient entry into the system can be done by interview if a terminal can be reserved for this purpose. When a terminal or an operator isn't available, new-patient registration can be accomplished using a source document. You must be consistent, though. It's not efficient to interview some patients and have others complete a form. If you need more information for collection purposes than what the computer program allows for input, a form definitely should be completed and kept as part of the permanent record.

CONSULTATIONS. For some medical practices, many new patients come from hospital consultations. Whenever a new patient is first seen outside the office, you must remember to bring the billing information back to the office. This helps to simplify office procedures. The information is usually obtainable directly from the patient's hospital chart. If your staff has to call the hospital for this information, there's a time lag before the information is entered into your system.

AUTHORIZATION FOR RELEASE OF DATA. If it's standard office procedure for patients to authorize the release of medical information to insurance companies, or to authorize the assignment of benefits to you on a special office form at the time of their initial visits, policy must be established for this to continue with the new system. As noted in Chapter 14, signature authorizations cannot be stored in the computer, but an automated system *can* print "signature on file." Of course, some carriers require that a copy of the signed authorization be attached to the form being submitted.

GETTING SIGNATURES FROM HOSPITALIZED PATIENTS. A policy also must be established for securing signatures from hospital patients. Should the form be mailed to them for completion, or should their signatures be obtained when they return to the office for follow-up care? If the latter, decide how the record will be flagged when it is entered into the computer so the staff will remember to secure the signature when the patient arrives.

Patient Account Status

With your new system in operation, the first function of each day—or the last function of the previous day—should be to inquire into the accounts of all the scheduled patients, to see if they've been paid or are currently being paid satisfactorily. This account check takes only a short time to accomplish, but gives you the opportunity to discuss payment of any past-due account while the patient is actually sitting across the desk from you.

If a statement has been returned in the mail as undeliverable, or if a patient hasn't been seen for a long time, the operator should notify the receptionist that she must update the patient's file by getting new information.

ON-LINE VERSUS BATCH PROCESSING. Many medical offices try to stay up to the minute with status information. Direct on-line posting updates accounts immediately. Batch processing updates them at the end of the function or the end of the day. This choice was, of course, an important consideration in shopping for your computer system. Whatever you have ended up with, you should set up your procedures to take maximum advantage of your system's capabilities.

Auditing Posted Charges

DAILY BALANCING. Charges to patients' accounts should be posted daily. The charge slips used for posting must balance with the computer total for charges posted. If there is a discrepancy, the error must be located and corrected.

To maintain accuracy, the charge slip amounts should be totaled on an adding machine or calculator and compared with the total charges listed on the computer-generated transaction journal report. If the totals don't agree, each posted transaction will have to be checked until the discrepancy is found. Then it must be corrected on the computer.

If a charge simply was not entered into the system, it must be posted before the operator can balance for the day. If an incorrect procedure was posted, a reversed entry will probably be necessary before the correct one can be entered. Never let an adjustment be entered to correct an error. And don't let daily totals be cleared from the computer system until the source documents' total has been balanced with the computer total.

OFFICE PATIENTS. The control system should be set up to verify that *all* charges for office patients are given to the business office every day. Prenumbered charge slips usually work well, as missing numbers can readily be determined. Having a list of the patients to be seen by each physician can also serve as a control system—there must be a charge slip for each patient. It's far easier to maintain a control system for office patients, of course, than for patients seen at other locations.

HOSPITAL CHARGES. Maintaining good control of patients' hospital charges can be difficult unless a systematic procedure is established to record them. If charges are held for posting following hospital discharge, all the procedures and charges for a patient's complete medical and/or surgical care can be entered into the computer, by dates. If admissions and daily charges are posted as they occur, statements rendered at the close of the billing cycle may be incomplete. For instance, if a patient is admitted to the hospital today and the first-day hospital charge is posted, and then tomorrow the billing cycle is closed and aged, a statement would be rendered for the first day of hospitalization. This would also cause the aging of the account for the same hospitalization to be split; the next cycle's statement would show the first-day charges to be 30 days old and the remaining hospital charges to be current. This is, of course, an undesirable situation.

CONTROLLING OUT-OF-OFFICE CHARGES. The computer can't process charges if physicians are lax in informing the office staff of all services rendered away from the office: emergency room visits, hospital admissions, consultations, diagnostic or surgical procedures, daily visits, and hospital discharges. This information should be given to the staff *daily*.

A reporting system is needed to help assure that out-of-office charges aren't being missed. The physicians must get in the habit of bringing back the ER sheets, consultation sheets, or other records, and regularly giving them to the right person. This is basically a matter of management and motivation of people. Without proper control and the cooperation of the physicians, it's difficult to maintain an effective system.

Bad business practices will defeat all the advantages that a computerized system has to offer. You can begin to see why a manual system with built-in problems—poor control, lack of communications, sloppy bookkeeping—will not be improved simply by wheeling in a computer.

Methods of Posting Payments

Payments can be posted to the system in either of two ways: indirectly, from a source document that summarizes the necessary data, or directly, from the checks and cash received daily for payment.

SOURCE DOCUMENT. It's probably wiser in the beginning to use a source document, at least until the operator is familiar with the system. But if you do, someone must complete the source document for data entry. When (and if) you graduate to the direct method, someone must be responsible for putting the patient's account number on each check for posting.

DIRECT METHOD. Putting the account number on the check will make it easy to key the entry into the right account. But if the payment should be posted to the wrong account, the error can be identified and corrected simply by tracking down a copy of the check with the correct account number on it. That way, you'd also know the check had been deposited.

VERIFICATION. Daily deposits must equal payments. Computer programs will generate bank deposit reports, or a summary of payments and adjustments, that reflect credits to patients' accounts. With even the best computer programs, though, controls must be established to verify the accuracy of the credits against the computer-generated report. These controls should include regular audits and double-checking. If there are discrepancies, the errors must be found and corrected.

Bank deposits should be made daily, to help ensure good accounting practices and to reduce the chances of embezzlement. The same person should never handle all the procedures for recording receipts. Division of duties helps to eliminate the misuse of funds and helps to provide better control of the cash flow.

CREDIT ADJUSTMENTS. There also must be control over credit adjustments to accounts. Otherwise, the door is wide open for fraud. A special source document must be used for a credit adjustment, or the computer system should be designed so that a credit adjustment cannot easily be entered into the system without verification (i.e., without appearing on daily printouts or audit trails).

File Maintenance

File maintenance allows for various patient-history data to be easily changed or corrected: for example, a change of address or telephone number, correction of date of birth, or change of primary and second-ary insurance carriers.

However, file maintenance *does not allow* other types of data to be changed with the same ease. Diagnosis and procedure codes, charges, payments, or credit/debit adjustments cannot be changed without a special procedure: For example, if the operator had posted an initial office visit (IOV) instead of a return visit to a patient's account—and charged $50 instead of $25—she would have to do a somewhat elabo-rate reversal (or backout) entry before posting the correct one. This is designed to prevent partial correction of errors, as well as to detect attempted fraud.

Adjustment of merely a financial error won't automatically adjust the rest of the incorrect information: procedure, diagnosis, location, and/ or physician. And backout or reversal procedures will always appear on the audit trails—and can be considered a warning flag requiring investigation by the computer administrator.

File maintenance involves the computer program's special sensitivity to certain fields (areas) within a record. It is an important software feature to look for in choosing your computer system.

Reports

Most computer systems allow for many kinds of reports to be gener-ated (see Chapter 19). The computer administrator not only must understand the purpose of these reports but also be able to interpret the information they generate, to use in auditing the system. The complexity of the business and the sophistication of the programs will determine what reports will be computer-generated and will become essential accounting records of your practice.

Audits in General

FREQUENCY. Audits are the only way to keep accurate records. Daily audits are the best way to detect mistakes, because they minimize the number of transactions reviewed per audit, and discrepancies can be found early.

Audits should also be performed monthly and annually, and may be necessary at other time intervals—quarterly, for instance. But if daily audits and controls are adequate, audits at longer intervals should merely substantiate the accuracy of your computer data.

OBJECTIVES. The primary objectives of audits for internal use are to test the effectiveness of the data processed, control of the information processed, and the efficiency of your operations.

CONTROL AREAS. For audits to be effective, the computer administrator should follow a checklist of control measures and items to review. The entries on the checklist would fall in three general areas: preventive, detective, and corrective.

Preventive. The task of the administrator in this area is to evaluate whether error-preventing measures are working effectively.

Detective. This area involves investigation of errors that do occur. The task is to analyze why errors are occurring and what can be done to eliminate them.

Corrective. In this area of control, the administrator makes sure that existing errors are being corrected *properly*, not just through some type of offset adjustment.

If everything in these control areas is properly followed and implemented by the computer administrator, your electronic data-processing business operation should be successful and your audits should be effective.

Independent Audits—a Must

Processing data through a computer does not eliminate the need for periodic independent audits. Your accountant, or his designee, should audit your system and the data in it. An independent audit must also evaluate the financial soundness of your business and the effectiveness of its internal controls. It is through audits that fraud can be detected or discouraged, performance reviewed, and accuracy of information determined.

You have the computer, you're on line, your data have been entered, and you're ready to go. But remember, continual auditing is the real key to a successful system.

17. Insurance Forms and Collections: Tough Tasks Made Easy

Your investment in the computer has been your most significant acknowledgment of the fact that your medical practice is, in fact, a business. And nothing is as critical to the operation of a business as maximizing payments, accounts receivable, and cash flow. The computer is here to help. And it will.

Speeding Up Insurance Claims

Automating your insurance claims processing will probably be the biggest single aid to improving income provided by the computer. We're living in an age of third-party payers, and you no doubt have the clerical workload to prove it.

You need an enormous amount of information to properly file claims, furnish the required patient signatures, do the record-keeping, follow up on actions, supply further information, answer questions, and know what questions to ask when problems arise.

If you don't file insurance claims on your patients' behalf, you still must furnish them with complete information relative to their medical treatment in a form acceptable to all the insurance carriers. Today, it takes a computer to deal with a computer; a computer is ideal for processing insurance claims and providing patients with whatever information they need.

How Computer-Generated Claims Are Processed

Computer-generated insurance claims can usually be processed daily, weekly, or whenever needed. They can also be processed individually or in batches, such as a week's worth of Medicare claims. The capability of your computer system determines how often claims are processed. Your computer should provide some form of control for keeping track of claims that have been generated and those that need to be generated. It's important to know what form of control you have.

INSURANCE CLAIM PERIOD. Your office, for example, may handle a small volume of insurance claims, so you've decided on weekly processing. The operator must enter the insurance period into the system. Since claim processing is done weekly, the insurance period will be changed weekly. The first week of operation would therefore be period 1 for insurance-processing purposes; the second week would be period 2, and so forth. The computer then tracks all transactions posted into each period. At the end of the week, the computer is instructed to generate all insurance claims for the transactions posted in period 1.

If all claims are processed on the universal claim form, the insurance claims can be generated quickly. If, however, insurance claims are generated by classifications, and special claim forms are used for each, it will be necessary to load the printer with the appropriate form before printing the claims for that class.

For instance, the operator will load Blue Shield claim forms into the printer and all Blue Shield claims for insurance period 1 will be printed. Then she'll load the printer with another special claim form and print all *those* claims for period 1, and so forth, until all the claims for each class have been produced. The insurance period will not be changed until all classes of claims for the current period have been printed.

CONTROL FOR TRACKING INSURANCE CLAIMS. With the kind of system we've been talking about, the computer keeps track of insurance claims by insurance periods only. In other words, it's the insurance period number assigned to a transaction that tells the computer whether or not an insurance claim has been processed for that transaction. Good management obviously dictates that *all* the claims in a given period be processed before the period is changed. Any exceptions would have to be tracked manually by the computer administrator. Having insurance forms completed for some but not all insurance classifications could undo your carefully constructed control network. Although a computer program of this type would probably allow for storage of some insurance periods as a precautionary measure, it's not wise to attempt splitting a period for any reason except an emergency.

DUPLICATE CLAIMS. Insurance periods must be changed promptly, whether daily, weekly, or biweekly. If the operator forgets to change the period, the computer will generate a duplicate claim for each of the claims previously processed for the period still entered in the system. Since human errors do occur, it's in your best interest to control for duplicate claims generation.

Duplicate claims must be caught *before* they're submitted to insurance carriers or patients. It takes human intervention and good management control to stop compounding the costs created by such errors. In order to institute management controls that will best mesh with the system, your computer administrator must be familiar with every business operation of your office as well as with the computer programs.

MAKE YOUR COMPUTER WORK FOR YOU. Although the above illustration may sound complicated, you have the flexibility and capability to make the system work for your practice. Some systems do not provide options. For example, insurance claims may be generated daily. The generation of claim forms is governed by posted procedures. Suppose you saw a patient for an office visit who has Medicare insurance. When the transaction is posted to the account, the computer reads the insurance data (the patient has Medicare insurance) and automatically generates the claim for the procedure performed. For hospital patients, the entry date for discharge may trigger the claim to be generated. The claims generated may go to spooler entries. Consequently, the only flexibility is controlled by the printing of the insurance forms. It's wise, however, to print all spooler entries on a daily basis for maintaining better control of the system. (Spooler entries can be deleted or lost should the system malfunction, and spooler entries have accidentally been deleted by human error.)

Is it wrong to consider a program of this type? Not necessarily. The quicker claims are processed, the faster the revenue should be forthcoming. It does demonstrate, however, that the computer will control your billing procedures. For instance, if it were necessary for you to see a patient on Monday and again on Friday, two insurance claims would be generated. You would not be able to process the claims on a weekly basis for both procedures to be printed on one claim form. The computer generates claims on a daily basis only.

Making the Process Efficient

YOUR PRINTER. Although a computer will generate insurance claims quickly, the overall process is only as fast as your printer. A printer that produces forms slowly, or one that's difficult to load and adjust, can significantly detract from efficiency. Obviously, if you don't use the universal claim form, your computer operator can spend a good deal of time loading and unloading the various classes of insurance forms.

PROGRAMMING FOR ALL SITUATIONS. It's impossible, of course, for a computer to generate more information on an insurance claim than has been processed into the system. The computer cannot do disability insurance, for example, if the program doesn't allow for it or if the dates for total and/or partial disability are not entered into it—even though the program allows for *storage* of this information. The system's output is governed both by input and by programmed instructions.

MANUAL SUPPORT. If the program doesn't allow for all types of insurance claims to be generated, or if it doesn't generate all of the required information for a claim to be processed, the system needs manual support: additional work to be performed after the insurance claims are printed. If you're accepting assignment of benefits from a particular patient, for example, it may be necessary to attach a copy of the patient's authorization. And some claims will need your signature or that of your authorized agent. However, your overall objective—to process all insurance claims accurately, efficiently, and promptly from start to finish—hasn't changed. To produce a successful result, manual operations must be well organized.

NEED FOR LEADERSHIP. To achieve this, the computer administrator must lead the way. Tasks must be assigned and time allocated for completing the various manual tasks. An organized staff should quickly accomplish the necessary work when each member understands her individual duties. Staffers should also understand that their efforts will turn productivity into revenue as rapidly as possible.

Without leadership, organization, and control, you'll likely have a disgruntled staff. People won't want to do the work, and the inevitable complaint will arise: *The computer isn't any good.* It's easier to do all the work by hand! Office assistants will do their worst to undermine the system, to prove it can't possibly work efficiently.

How will you overcome their resistance? By emphasizing how quickly the computer works, and how "willing" it is to do the repetitious, detailed work that staff members find so tedious.

The speed may frighten your office staff at first. The computer can generate claims so rapidly that your assistants may be afraid they can't keep up. But generated claims that pile up on a desk for days before final manual preparation are costly—indicative of poor management control and lack of planning. Don't blame the computer for office inefficiencies. It did its work when it printed the claims. Make sure your assistants understand the importance of following through.

PAPERLESS CLAIMS. Claims transmitted electronically are paperless claims. If your computer is compatible with the computer used by the insurer, it is actually possible to submit claims on magnetic tape, or by telephone hookup using a modem. There are several advantages to this—speed, efficiency, accuracy, greater likelihood of transmitting all pertinent information—and it is worthwhile investigating. To determine compatibility, consult your insurance carriers, especially the high-volume ones such as Blue Shield and Medicare.

Insurance claims, of course, make up only a part of your accounts billing. You still have to improve collections for the rest of your receivables, and the computer will surely help you here, too.

Improving Your Collections

Depending on your specialty and area of the country, your accounts receivable should equal, on average, one to three months' gross charges, and your collection ratio should be at least 90 percent. Have you been achieving this with your old manual system?

Decreasing the age of your accounts receivable and increasing collections will not be difficult with your new computer system . . . *if* you and your staff develop and implement effective procedures to strengthen the collection process. For starters, by helping your office run more efficiently and doing much of the drudgery, the computer will allow your employees more time for better use of their resources, including collections. However, a computer can do much more to upgrade your collection system.

Itemized Statements

The first step in obtaining payment is to render an itemized statement listing the medical care or procedures performed. Statements must be legible, accurate, and timely. They must also be mailed promptly.

Preparing statements is an annoying, time-consuming chore in most medical offices. Often the telephone rings for several days after statements have gone out because of errors in accounting. In some offices, not all statements are mailed on a regular basis and account balances are not aged. Manually controlling the accounts receivable is a difficult task at best.

Computer-generated statements, on the other hand, permit better control of accounts receivable because they are accurate, thorough, legible, and timely. A computer-generated statement resembles a typewritten statement; it's easy to read. It itemizes the services rendered during the billing period, and should age any previous outstanding balance. As an account ages, the computer will also generate an appropriate message calling attention to the delinquency. Telephone calls inquiring about errors on accounts should be virtually eliminated. Furthermore, computer-generated statements will go out regularly and on time. The end result: better control of the accounts receivable, increased collections, and a decrease in outstanding accounts.

The Multipurpose Billing Form

One way the computer can help decrease billing problems is by producing a multipurpose billing form (Fig. 17-1). Such a billing form is usually designed in triplicate: two copies to the patient—one for his records, the other for submission to his insurance carrier; the third copy is retained by the medical office. Because the billing form is handed to the patient as he checks out at the desk following his visit, it's hoped it will encourage payment at that time.

If the patient does not pay in full at the time of service, a self-addressed return envelope can be provided with the multipurpose billing form, along with a request that payment for the balance be mailed to the office. If the system works, the costs involved in mailing statements will be greatly reduced. So, too, will the need to process insurance claims. The medical information the patient needs to file his own claim is right on the billing form; the patient merely attaches it to his insurance form.

Data Mailers

Data mailers are itemized statements, self-contained for mailing. They're similar to multipurpose billing forms, except they're designed to be mailed. If your data mailers include self-addressed return envelopes, the statement and envelope will be enclosed in another sealed envelope—addressed to the patient—with any outstanding balances on account noted. If the program allows for it, automatic messages can be printed on delinquent accounts.

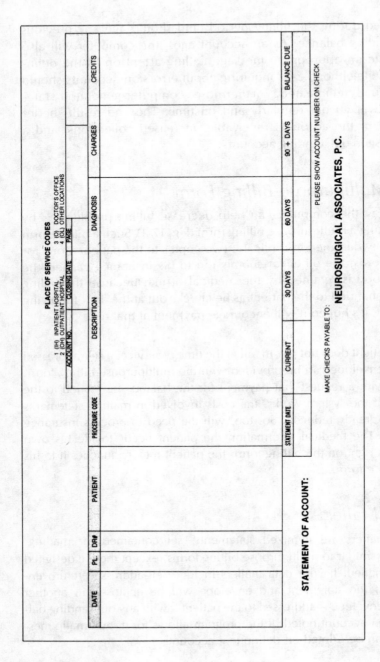

Figure 17.1. An example of a multipurpose billing form, an itemized statement with supporting codes difining diagnosis, procedures, place of service, etc. It is usually accepted by insurance companies as proof of service in lieu of a completed claim form.

Postal information (first-class presort mail, forwarding address re-quested, and permit imprints) can be printed on the outside envelope. Since there are rules and regulations governing the printing of this information, consult the U.S. Postal Service first.

SORTING AND MAILING. Data mailers come off the computer in con-tinuous form, but can quickly be separated if they're perforated. If your volume is large enough to qualify for first-class presort mail, postage is cheaper, but the statements must be sorted according to ZIP codes. Since many programs print data mailers according to ZIP code se-quence anyway, this should present no problem and can be done easily. To find out whether or not you qualify for first-class presort rates, contact the Postal Service.

MAILING SCHEDULE. Although many consultants recommend mailing statements around the first of the month, it's far more important to develop a schedule for rendering and mailing them at *regular intervals.* A computer can provide the control for this.

Not all statements need to be mailed on the same day of the month. You can set up billing cycles that spread the job out evenly instead of concentrating all the work into a few days every month.

Cycle Billing

With cycle billing, accounts receivable are divided into roughly equal segments by alphabetical or financial classification, for instance, and each week one segment is prepared for the mail.

ALPHABETICAL DIVISION. If your accounts are divided alphabet-ically, all patients whose names begin with A through G might be billed during the first week of the month, H through M the second week, N through S the third week, and T through Z the fourth. Easy enough. But if the N-to-S segment, for example, is twice the size of the T-to-Z group, you'll have to reapportion, as the point is to send out roughly the same number of statements each week. Also, mailing dates should remain constant to within the nearest working day.

DIVISION ACCORDING TO FINANCIAL CLASSIFICATION. Instead of dividing your accounts alphabetically, you can divide them according to source of payment: Blue Shield, Medicare, commercial insurance, workers' compensation, welfare, self-pay, and so on. Here again, the accounts must be divided as evenly as possible to distribute the work of billing and mailing evenly throughout the month.

The advantage of this method is that it makes it easy to evaluate the effectiveness of collections from the various sources of payment, since the computer has already broken down your accounts that way. You may then decide on different write-off or adjustment policies according to financial classification.

DAILY CYCLE BILLING. Some systems generate bills automatically on a daily basis. You tell the computer when you want to bill the patient: for example, 10 days following treatment. Since patients and procedures are keyed into the system on a daily basis, statements begin to generate on a daily basis and then on the same date each month thereafter until the account zeroes out. With this type of system, the computer controls the billing procedures. Since statements should be mailed promptly, you may not qualify for special postal discount rates for bulk mail. On the other hand, it may be easier for your staff to prepare the statements for mail on a daily basis, particularly if data mailers are not used. The computer also would automatically age your accounts receivable.

Special Accounts

Some accounts don't require statements—Medicaid accounts, accounts that have gone to a collection agency, and courtesy accounts, for example. Your program should allow for such accounts to be specially coded to prevent the generation of a statement. The code would tell the computer to put these accounts on "hold" status and indicate the reason: code 1 could signify a patient who receives professional courtesy; code 2 might mean a bad address; code 3 could flag those accounts on which you accept insurance as payment in full.

It's also important to be able to release accounts from "hold" status at any time. Finally, make one person responsible for overseeing special accounts and their codes.

A Word About Collection Agencies

Collection agencies are not entitled to—and should not be given— information relative to diagnosis and treatment. Even if the information is encoded, don't assume it can't be deciphered. So be careful when giving any computer printouts to a collection agency; they may contain legally tricky information.

With a computer system, of course, you should have less need to turn accounts over to a collection agency anyway.

Aging Analysis Report

Before each new billing cycle, the current cycle must be closed and aged. This is easily accomplished by entering a command into the system that generates an accounts receivable aging analysis report. The report ages the balance of the accounts receivable into: current, 30 days, 60 days, 90 days, and so on. Some systems will automatically age your accounts receivable, but you need to understand how it's accomplished.

This information is important to the collection process. To have it and not use it is simply a waste of paper—and money. Your practice must have a firm collections policy, and enforce it by means of "overdue" notices on statements, collection letters, telephone calls, and, finally, submission of delinquent accounts to a collection agency.

Monthly Financial Reports

At the close of every month there are special instructions to be followed, and someone—the computer administrator—needs to be responsible for carrying out the necessary work. The financial totals for month-to-date will shift to year-to-date, and all monthly activities will be closed.

Monthly reports will be generated and can be used to help spot problems as they occur—before you feel the major effects. For example, suppose the revenue received from Blue Shield is extremely low, as compared to other months. Is it because (1) your staff has not been processing the claims, (2) your claim rejection rate is exceedingly high, or (3) you're seeing more patients with Medicaid insurance and fewer patients who have Blue Shield coverage? A high rejection rate may indicate poor information management; perhaps you need to enroll some staff members in a Blue Shield workshop as quickly as possible. If you don't correct the problem on a timely basis, the effects usually become more severe.

In summary, a computer provides the information needed for management and control, but it takes people to interpret the information for administering sound management and control to help ensure the success of your business operations.

There's an old saying that "he who controls the data controls the company." Have you ever thought about why software vendors offer management services? They know what to do with the information provided by the computer. Someone must be administratively responsible for the success of your operations.

18. Accounting: You'll Welcome This Addition

A general ledger program is considered a luxury for most small businesses. But if you can justify the purchase of one, you'll find your computer has bookkeeping capabilities that open up a world of attractive features.

The General Ledger Program

The system uses a "ledger" to classify business transactions by accounts. It houses all of your assets, liabilities, and capital accounts. By posting transactions—income or expense—to these accounts, it calculates and records increases and decreases. The general ledger also provides a history of transactions affecting your assets, liabilities, and income during the calendar or fiscal year.

INCOME AND EXPENSE RECORD. The computer with a general ledger program can maintain a daily record of all income and expenditures—checking account deposits, bills paid, checks written, and so on. It can, in fact, keep your entire checking account for you—recording checks, balancing statements, even printing certain checks.

CLASSIFICATION OF EXPENSES. The computer may even be able to keep track of whether checks are written for deductible business expenses (for example, payroll, supplies, fire and theft coverage), depreciable capital expenses (the computer, if you purchase it!), or nondeductible expenses (disability insurance premiums, your family's travel expenses to a medical convention).

You may also be able to program your computer to keep track of personal expenses. However, most practice management consultants feel it's unwise to spend office funds for personal uses. And if you're incorporated, the IRS will frown on this habit.

DEBIT AND CREDIT MEMOS. Occasionally, you receive debit memos or credit memos from the bank. You get a debit memo when a bad check is included in one of your deposits, for example, or when you're charged for check printing or a monthly service fee. The general ledger system will automatically deduct that amount from your balance; it doesn't write it down on a scrap of paper and then forget to transfer it onto your checkbook register. If it's a bad check from a patient that causes the debit memo, the computer will also automatically debit the amount on the patient's ledger card.

Credit memos are less common. Your assistant may have made a mistake in filling out the deposit slip—or the bank may have made an error. Again, the computer will automatically adjust your account and bring your balance up to date.

TRANSFER OF TAX DATA. At the end of the year, the computer should be able to transfer all your transaction records, income, capital-expense, and operating-expense statements, and tax reports out of the active file to make room for the coming year's records. Tax reports should be transferred to a holding file until your return is prepared and submitted to the IRS. Any other data held beyond this time can be stored in the computer's memory bank, or printed during off hours, and filed as part of your paper records for as long as you need.

Capital Expenses

When expenditures are posted to the expense ledger accounts, the computer will automatically post certain items to the capital equipment and improvement account. Expenses for equipment—such as a new file cabinet, microscope, tables for the waiting room, labor charges for remodeling—are all posted to this account. Obviously, the amounts will vary from month to month; there may be no entries at all in some months.

EQUIPMENT INFORMATION. When an amount is posted to a capital account, the computer may also be programmed to itemize, on the income and expenditure account, when the purchase was made, the total price, model number, serial number, sales tax, number of the check or checks used to pay for it, and so forth. If the equipment came from one of the manufacturers or suppliers your practice does a lot of business with, you can assign the supplier a code number, which the computer will also apply to the transaction.

PAYMENT SCHEDULE. The computer will also take into account the payment schedule. If it's a major purchase, the basis will likely be 30-60-90: one-fourth of the price paid on delivery, one-fourth in a month, one-fourth at two months, and the final quarter after three months. The computer will then produce a payment memo at each interval—or the check itself—and will update the balance due.

YEAR-END REPORT. At the end of each year, the computer will prepare a recapitulation of all equipment and improvement entries shown in the ledger. All information regarding model numbers, serial numbers, manufacturers, guarantees, and repair service will be posted as well. Have two copies prepared: an office copy and one to be forwarded to your accountant.

DEPRECIATION SCHEDULES. Capital expenses aren't tax-deductible; instead, they're depreciable. For every piece of equipment you buy and every improvement you contract for, determine the number of years over which you want to write it off. With a general ledger program, the computer will enter depreciation as an operating expense for tax purposes.

Accounts-Payable Program

The computer should be able to track unpaid suppliers' bills and process payments either on a periodic basis (such as monthly) or whenever the bills come in. The computer maintains an invoice log, which keeps a running list of charges, returns, payments, and credits. The date of purchase, the supplier's charge number, the date of the bill, and the amount owed are all kept on file, as well as any returns or shortages of items delivered.

When a supplier's monthly statement arrives, it's keyed into the computer and the computer checks it against the information it already has on file. If the data and the invoice agree, the computer will so indicate and may then punch out a check in payment of the bill. This can be especially efficient when a number of bills all come in at once, such as around the first of the month. It will also prove efficient when, as all too commonly happens, balances are wrong or in dispute, letters pass in the mail, payments are not credited, interest charged is incorrect, and so forth.

Payroll

Having your office payroll on the computer can be a valuable supplement to the accounts-payable program. Payroll checks will be computer-generated, and so will reports for Social Security (FICA), federal tax withholding, state tax withholding, and any other money withheld from employees' pay.

Each employee must fill out a new W-4 form, entering full name, Social Security number, address, marital status, and number of withholding exemptions claimed. There will also be space for employees to request withholding for your practice's corporate or Keogh pension or profit-sharing plan or their own individual retirement accounts.

As payday nears, the computer should update each employee's salary record for both the current pay period and the calendar year (according to federal requirements). It will then produce the paycheck.

The computer should keep track of both cumulative and current regular earnings, any overtime, federal, state, and city withholding, FICA taxes, and any other withholding (outstanding loans, unpaid leaves of absence, employee-paid insurance policies, and the like). It will periodically add up all these totals—weekly, monthly, quarterly, or just annually—and keep a running record for each staff member.

The speed, accuracy, and flexibility of the program will make life easier for your staff. They'll no longer have to recalculate payroll data every time the tax rate changes, or an employee adds or subtracts an exemption.

The computer will also generate quarterly reports for tax purposes, and W-2 forms at year-end.

Cost-Effectiveness

A general ledger program can be extremely valuable for a large medical practice, but it's usually costly and may be difficult to justify for a smaller one.

What will it do for you? It should be able to give you financial statements, balance sheets, profit and loss statements, and other accounting services. It can total and balance all ledgers on a daily, weekly, monthly, or quarterly basis, and locate any posted errors before they become critical.

It can keep track of all income, itemize all operating expenses (office and medical supplies, payroll, insurance, rent, utilities, dues and subscriptions, licenses, taxes, and so on), depreciate your capital expenditures, and balance the whole thing each month.

SIZE OF YOUR PRACTICE. If you're wondering whether this is for you, start by comparing the size of your operation versus the cost of a program like this. But also consider to what extent your staff keeps putting all these time-consuming tasks off, and to what extent you're hampered by financial reports that are completed too late to be of much use to you.

COMPARISON WITH OUTSIDE SERVICES. If you use an accountant or other outside service to perform much of your practice's accounting and bookkeeping, balance this cost against the cost of purchasing or leasing the hardware and software capability of performing the same functions in-office.

(A computer can't entirely replace your accountant. You'll always need someone thoroughly versed in the tax laws to guide you and your staff in operating the business side of your practice. But it's certainly possible for a computer to take over the menial tasks and lengthy calculations you may have been paying your accountant a premium to perform for you—in all probability, on a computer of his own.)

Meeting Government Reporting Requirements

One of the biggest advantages of a computerized accounting system could be the way in which it processes all income and earning reports required by the IRS.

FORM 941. The quarterly 941 form, for example, must be filed with the IRS at the end of every March, June, September, and December. It must show, among other things, the total wages and tips subject to withholding, plus other employee compensation; the total income tax withheld from wages, tips, pensions, annuities, sick pay, etc.; the taxable FICA wages paid; the total FICA taxes; net taxes; and the record of federal tax liability. Then any taxes due or overpayments made must be computed, and a check must be processed to accompany the form for any balance owed.

This is an imposing task to perform manually every three months. The computer, however, can spew the information from its data base almost instantaneously, can even print it right onto the forms, and can produce the check as well.

UNEMPLOYMENT INSURANCE TAXES. Another big obligation is the unemployment insurance reports, both federal and state.

To prepare the state unemployment tax report manually, for example, your bookkeeper must go through no fewer than 11 time-consuming steps . . . for each employee. The computer, on the other hand, can

generate the same report in minutes. Furthermore, mistakes are practically impossible.

FORMS W-2 AND W-3. Finally, every employer must complete a W-2
form (federal wage and tax statement) at the end of every year for each
employee. Filling out the statement may not be a burden. But culling
all the information from the previous 12 months and totaling it for each
employee might be.

In addition, accompanying all the W-2s sent to the IRS must be one
W-3 form, on which must be entered:

1. Your state identification number
2. The number of W-2 forms enclosed (one for each current and ex-
   employee)
3. The date of the report
4. Total FICA tax withheld
5. Total federal income tax withheld
6. Total FICA wages
7. Total wages, tips, and other compensation
8. Your federal identification number
9. Your name, address, and ZIP code
10. Your signature and the date.

An office with two doctors and three employees might have no trouble
manually producing the W-2 and W-3 forms. One with six doctors and
10 or more employees, on the other hand, might consider the advantages of having the computer produce them.

FORM 940. Finally, every medical practice must annually prepare a
940 form—the employer's annual federal unemployment tax return.
Form 940 is a recapitulation of the amount of unemployment tax
you've already paid to the state fund, plus a computation of the federal
unemployment tax.

The computations can get very time-consuming and tricky for employees whose eyelids become heavy as they pore over the figures between
handling patients in the midst of a heavy day, during lunch hour, or

whenever else they can fit the work in. The computer has no eyelids— or lunch hours.

Any one of these jobs may not, in itself, be enough to justify the purchase of a general ledger program. But if you have a system in-house, these are some of the ways it can make your life easier.

19. Reports: If You Can Think of One, Your Computer Can Probably Provide It

The aging analysis report of accounts receivable discussed in Chapter 17 and the tax reports discussed in Chapter 18 are only some of the many reports a computer can generate. In fact, whatever is entered into the system should be able to be retrieved from it. But since programs don't necessarily plan for the formatted retrieval of *all* information, modifications may have to be made to produce reports of exactly the information you desire. Modifications usually are costly, however, so it's always better to acquire software in the beginning that has just the features that suit your needs.

Some reports are essential to the accounting process and represent mandatory financial records; others may just contain useful information. Careful: With a computer system, it's easy to become inundated with paper. If some of the available reports aren't actually used, don't print them! Generate only the reports that are essential and/or beneficial to your practice.

You must also determine how often each kind of report is needed: daily, weekly, monthly, quarterly, semiannually, or annually. Finally, you must decide which reports must be kept and filed and which can be viewed and destroyed.

Audit Trails of Accounts Receivable

Audit trails of charges are reports essential for accounting purposes. They're records of the transactions affecting accounts receivable and represent *potential* earned income. Audit trails of payments and adjustments, on the other hand, represent *actual* earned income.

Financial Statements

Financial statement reports may show charges, payments, and adjustments on a daily, month-to-date, and year-to-date basis. These totals may be reported by financial classifications, alpha cycle billing, office location, doctor, or any combination of these factors that's relevant to your business operation. Financial statements may be long and comprehensive or short and specialized. Either way, they provide information essential to your business decisions.

Patient Master File Report

A patient master file report may be needed at any time. It's simply a list of all the patients' accounts on the computer (*not* a list of all patients ever seen in the office). In implementing your new system, you'll have started by entering only the current accounts receivable and will have added other accounts only as patients returned. You should not attempt to add all back accounts into the computer system. However, you'll still want to run and check the patient master file report periodically just to verify its accuracy.

When the computer is running as a stand-alone system (see Chapter 20), you'll have to decide how often to generate a patient master file report. As long as the computer is up and running, there's not much need for it. But if the computer goes down for an extended period, the report becomes useful.

Accounts Receivable Aging Analysis

The accounts receivable aging analysis report should be run monthly, either at the time of cycle billing of each segment or at the time of monthly billing of the entire account, as discussed in Chapter 17. This report should print all the necessary information for telephoning or contacting patients to discuss balances due. Your assistant should not need additional information or have to consult medical charts.

CYCLE BILLING. If cycle billing is done weekly, the aging analysis report may list only the accounts on that cycle. This provides better control of delinquent accounts, because it allows your staff to work the accounts throughout the month for a better collection ratio. Work can also be distributed more evenly; a different staff member might be responsible for each cycle's collections.

BREAKDOWN OF ACCOUNTS BY AGE. Whether you bill monthly or cycle-bill, you should be able to print out a complete listing of accounts receivable at any given time. This is especially useful at the close of each month. This report may reveal other important information, such as the percentage value of the aged receivables relative to the total balance due. For example, your accounts can be aged out to 90 days, and their total dollar value shown as equaling 100 percent. The dollar amounts in the various columns for aging account balances (30 days, 60 days, 90 days, and current) would be totaled, and the total in each category would be computed as a percentage of the 100 percent grand total.

This is valuable information. The older an account balance becomes, the less likely it is to be collected; the older the balance, in other words, the larger the loss of income (see Chapter 3).

In addition to the overall aging analysis report, you may be able to obtain special aging analysis reports, such as a listing of all accounts 60 days old and/or with a balance of $100 or more.

OTHER STATISTICAL INFORMATION. The accounts receivable aging analysis report may reveal other statistical information. You may ask for a printout of the total number of accounts according to each source of payment, listing the outstanding dollar balance for each source and the percentage relative to the total accounts receivable.

This kind of analysis can give you important information about your collections. For example, it may reveal that most of your patients' accounts are classified as covered by commercial insurance but the largest outstanding balance is for accounts covered by Blue Shield. What might this tell you? That Blue Shield claims are not being filed promptly, that they're being filed incorrectly, or that there's no follow-up on your staff's part. Good information to have.

PURGING. The report may also tell you the total number of accounts in the computer, including the number of zero-balance accounts. Zero-balance accounts aren't necessarily inactive. But after an inactive account has been kept on the computer for a certain period of time—a year, say—you may want to have it purged to make room for new accounts. When accounts are purged from the system, they must be stored in some other medium. It may simply be hard copy—a printout of the account and all the transactions recorded on it—or it may be microfilm.

Diagnoses/Procedures Reports

Many systems can generate reports based on diagnoses and procedures. These reports may reveal only the number of patients treated per diagnosis; or they may show the yearly revenue per procedure; or they may even list all the patients between the ages of 20 and 35 who were treated for hypertension within the past year.

This kind of analysis can be valuable for clinical research as well as for running the business side of your practice.

Using Reports

We've reviewed a few of the types of reports your computer system may be able to provide. In general, all reports provide information. The value of this information depends on how you interpret it and how you act on your interpretation. The computer cannot do this for you. It can only help point the way.

20. The Computer Stands Alone

Audits and Controls

Before the computer is accepted as the only accounting system for accounts receivable, the system's soundness and accuracy must be tested. An audit of your old manual system against the new computerized one will help ensure this. Chapter 15 went into the advantages and disadvantages of parallel processing versus the "guts" method of conversion. But the only way you'll know for sure whether your new computer can stand alone is to have an audit performed.

An audit is usually thought of as an official examination and verification of account books or an accounting system performed by a certified public accountant. But this definition isn't totally correct. That's because there are really two types of audits: an attest audit and an operational audit.

Attest Audit

Very briefly, an attest audit provides the basis for expression of an opinion on financial statements. It must almost always be performed by a certified public accountant, who determines whether the financial reports of a business or other entity have been prepared according to "generally accepted accounting procedures." The CPA's opinion is acceptable as legal evidence; in fact, attest audits are often done to satisfy legal requirements.

You'll leave attest audits to your accountant, pretty much as you've done in the past. What we're more concerned with here is the operational audit.

Operational Audit

The operational audit is an internal audit. When correctly done, it can reliably assess the correctness of your automated accounting procedures as well as the efficiency, cost-effectiveness, and security of your new data-processing system.

WHO AND WHEN. Your computer administrator should be in charge of your practice's operational audits. Especially at first, she and you may wish to involve your accountant. Once your administrator fully understands what's required and has established a routine, however, the accountant should be able to bow out of the picture.

Operational audits can be performed as often—or as seldom—as circumstances dictate for your business office. In the beginning, it may be a good idea for you to sit down with your partner(s), your office manager and computer administrator, and your accountant and decide how often to audit your business operations internally. As time passes and everyone gains familiarity with the computer, however, you'll probably want to change the frequency of these regular audits.

CONTROL OF THE OPERATION. In a small practice, one person might effectively control the entire computer operation. If that person became ill—or went on vacation—your computer functions could come to a screeching halt. If she suddenly quit, you could be in real trouble. That's why you should always have a backup—even if you're the only one available.

In a larger practice, even with several computer operators, it still wouldn't hurt if at least one of the doctors had more than passing knowledge about the computer system. And where several computer operators are utilized, their duties must be separated according to good accounting and control procedures.

SEPARATION OF RESPONSIBILITIES. An arrangement whereby anyone can enter any information into the system at any time invites mischief. You don't have to go so far as the "fail-safe" procedures reputed to govern missile firing, but the underlying principles of security are really the same.

First, certain kinds of information should be acceptable to the computer only under certain conditions. For example, the computer may be programmed to reject input of today's accounts receivable until yesterday's file has been verified and closed.

Second, don't entrust any one office assistant—let alone all of them—with access to every computer function. No matter how much you trust your staff, you must recognize that fraud can—and does—happen in some medical offices, both large and small. So keep every employee from becoming so familiar with the system that she's tempted to go into business for herself.

HEADING OFF EMBEZZLEMENT. With your manual system, it was easy enough to spot a written account card that had been altered. Your employees knew, too, how easy it would be to spot—as long as you were reasonably vigilant. But with a computer system, a clever operator can alter numbers, and it can be quite difficult to follow the tracks. Even if you happen to spot something that doesn't seem quite right to you, it can be tough to confirm your suspicions. If you question an employee you feel may be manipulating figures on the computer, she's likely to tell you: "I don't know, Doctor. This darn machine . . ." Yet she may know very well.

Having your office manager or computer administrator in charge gives you a way of fixing responsibility. If there's any discrepancy, she should be able to track it down. One feature that should be a part of your system is an "exceptions" report. This report prints out any adjustments or write-offs in billing entered by an employee. A code identifies the employee who entered the exception, and the report should be available only to the office manager or computer administrator and you.

WHO WATCHES THE WATCHERS? In the computer era, the answer to this age-old question is: your CPA. Through periodic attest audits, your accountant should be able to catch evidence of any fraud on the part of your office manager or computer administrator—or, for that matter, the doctors themselves. If you have any reason to suspect fraud, of course, you can always call your accountant in for some immediate detective work.

MANUAL CHECKS. In addition to the operational audit, you might want to set up other methods of cross-checking figures. For example, you might try batching the daysheets, then running control tapes for a certain period, comparing these tapes with the totals on the computer, and then comparing those totals with the computer's regular reports. Here again, you'll have to be willing to get involved.

DISASTER PREVENTION AND RECOVERY. In addition to assessing security and management control, the operational audit should include disaster prevention and recovery—that is, system backup. If disaster (total or partial loss of stored data) should occur, are your records protected by a backup medium? How difficult would it be to get your accounting system back into operation following a disaster? Would any of the completed work have to be repeated? Does your backup procedure provide the protection that's necessary to begin recovery right at the point where the disaster occurred? You must have satisfactory answers to all these questions!

Remember that once you've computerized your office, just about the entire welfare of your practice is in that machine. Your whole practice is sitting on that storage disk, vulnerable to a foul-up by a data-entry clerk or one of your vendor's (possibly low-paid) programmers.

BACKING UP YOUR DISK. Don't let a foul-up sink you. Make a copy of your disk pack every day. Every decent software package provides the capability. You simply copy the computer data to the backup media by entering a few simple commands. Then you take the backup media to some safe place. Ideally, it should be placed in a fire-proof safe.

It's good to use a three- or four-tier "son-father-grandfather-great grandfather" backup system. For example, if your backup media is onto tape, tonight you would backup onto the tape you call the son. Tomorrow you backup onto a different tape called the father. The next day you backup onto a third tape called the grandfather. The fourth day you backup onto the fourth tape called the great grandfather. The fifth day you backup onto the son again.

The reason for all this effort? Suppose something happens at the end of a day to wipe out your disk storage: a software problem, a power failure, anything. Your data have been destroyed—yet you don't know that this has happened. You back up, and you're copying a "corrupted" disk pack. Now your backup media is bad and you're in real trouble. You'll discover the problem the next morning when you try to operate your system. The problem, software or hardware, can be fixed. But your data are gone forever.

But with the son-father-grandfather backup system, you can get the great grandfather problem fixed, then use the most recently backed-up media and resume business. The most you could lose would be one or two days' data—never your entire files. The extra cost for the additional backup media may well be a wise trade-off for the redundant security.

Your computer administrator should take charge of disk backup, since she's the one who is basically responsible for security. She must know the system inside and out in order to maintain control over the overall operation.

Special Points of Control

Your computer operation must include specific control points to prevent errors. If errors occur—and they will—they must be found. Depending on what's being processed, attention to the control points should narrow down the fields for locating errors.

DATA VERIFICATION. When data are being entered, most programs give the operator a chance for correction by asking, in one form or another, "Data correct?" If the operator acknowledges that the data are, in fact, correct, the information is locked into the system and cannot be routinely changed. If the operator has made an incorrect entry and answers No, the program allows for the information to be corrected right then. This is a preventive control provided by the computer's software.

BACKING OUT. While it should be relatively easy to correct an error, it should be much more than a simple operation to change a transaction once it's locked into the system. Take, for example, a charge transaction, recorded at the time of the office visit, and the follow-up entry made when payment is received. This information should *not* be easy to change!

It should be necessary for the entire transaction to be backed out of the system (reversed) before any correction is made. The complete operation must be visible (appearing, for example, on the audit trails and exceptions report). If a $20 charge was recorded and then backed out, you need to know why. The backout may have been for a good reason—perhaps it was posted to the wrong physician—but there may be no good reason at all. When your computer software includes such a backout system, you're more likely to become aware of anything suspicious. Then you (or your computer administrator) can investigate and take any necessary action.

CONFIDENTIAL PASSWORDS. Another security function of the computer administrator is establishing a confidential file of operators' passwords, associating them with the functions each person is allowed to perform. The computer administrator should regularly change the passwords, and promptly delete those of departing employees.

BACKUP PERSONNEL SUPPORT. There should be a specific plan for backup support of the data-processing personnel. Illness should never prevent necessary work from being done. And specific, clearly written instructions should be available for backing up the disk for safe storage at day's end, just in case the person who regularly does this is out of the office. This is essential for keeping the business of the practice in operation if disaster should occur.

EVALUATING THE AUDIT. The internal (operational) audit will, of course, point up any deficiencies in security, as well as in accuracy, effectiveness, and control. But you and your colleagues should also emphasize to your staff the positive factors the audit uncovers.

Share the good as well as the bad with those involved in the data-processing operation. To focus on only the negative points will naturally produce negative feelings. But if you temper the bad news with good news, you'll find that your staff will be willing to work with you to solve the problems. It won't hurt morale, either, if you assure the staff that the new system is working—and that they're a major reason why it is!

During the period of parallel processing—manual and computer—there was probably so much work that there was a time lag in entering and processing data. But now the system should become more effective and the personnel more efficient. The computer will remain "new" for quite a while, and the staff will be constantly learning. By this time, though, your assistants should have overcome their initial fears and should be ready for going it alone with the computer.

Data-Processing Organization and Management—as Important as Your Software

The organization of the daily, weekly, and monthly work to be accomplished on the computer will ultimately help determine the success of the system—and your business operations. If parallel processing was continued until a consistent and accurate method was established, an important objective was achieved. Now it is time for other objectives to be accomplished in order to reach your long-range goals for your office computer system.

Communicating With Your Staff

To create a structure that allows your personnel to work comfortably with electronic data processing is not a simple task. But it can be achieved by organizing the work flow and listening to your people.

The cooperation of your employees will continue to be an essential element. The best way to get this cooperation is through good communication. There should always be an open door between management—you and your colleagues—and your staff. And your data-processing people should communicate with the rest of the staff, too. An exchange of problems and ideas can only work to your benefit. Your computer administrator or office manager will be a key to this approach. There are many methods she can use to enhance communication, and all will work—as long as she puts time and effort into it.

PERIODIC SYSTEM EVALUATIONS. In the early days of the stand alone phase of your computer operation, the people who work with the system will begin to evaluate their results. Their input could be vital, so you should constantly evaluate the information they pass along. As you create a comfortable atmosphere that allows for personal job growth, evaluations can become less frequent. But they will always be essential to keep up with changes affecting delivery of health care. Any changes that directly affect you usually affect your medical office and business operations.

UNDERSTANDING RESPONSIBILITIES AND GOALS. The success of the business side of your practice is dependent on every employee. Each one must understand her individual responsibilities and assignments. It's your job to make every employee aware of the overall goals of your medical practice—and how each of them fits into the scheme.

STAFF MEETINGS. Staff meetings provide the best opportunity for open communication. Here's where you can let down your hair—and let everyone else do the same. This is where both buck privates and generals should have their say without fear of repercussions. Directions can be given and plans and procedures discussed. The staff can let you and the other physicians know about problems they are seeing in their encounters with patients. Practical and effective solutions should be sought. The goal: providing your patients with the best possible medical care *and* the best possible services.

Whatever techniques are employed to effectively communicate, they should help strengthen the relationships between employer and employees. With everyone working in cooperation toward the same objectives, your goals will be easier to attain.

KEEPING PATIENTS HAPPY. The most direct effect that your employees can have on your practice involves their relations with patients. If patients aren't given prompt, courteous service—hopefully with a friendly smile—they'll look elsewhere for medical services. Competition among physicians is constantly growing; you should be competitive. Keep in mind that your patients are your most effective public relations tool.

PEOPLE ARE THE KEY. This discussion has emphasized three basic points: (1) physicians and medical assistants must constantly strive to meet the needs of patients, (2) the total success of your business operation depends on every employee, and (3) the overall goals of your practice must be clearly defined by you and understood by your staff. These points clearly demonstrate that *people* make the biggest contribution to the success of any medical practice. The computer is only a tool that can enhance business operations; this should be emphasized to everyone.

JOB DESCRIPTIONS. Effective personnel management is essential to an efficient computer operation. And written job descriptions are essential to effective personnel management. These should not only define each employee's duties, but also provide ongoing direction. With such guidance, conflicts should be reduced and a proper chain of command established. Merely introducing a computer system into your office will dictate the need for updated job descriptions for all employees. But don't foster a "that's not my job" syndrome by too strictly defining each area of responsibility. Stress the importance of mutual help. When a staff functions together as a smoothly running team, patients are almost guaranteed the best possible services.

Job descriptions should be a vital link to successful communication. But when implementing a computer system, it often takes a while before job descriptions can be updated or rewritten. Until then—and even after job descriptions are completed—the basic organizational structure of your office should be designed to enhance give-and-take.

Since communication is a two-way street, make sure you listen if you also want to be heard. If you and the other leaders in your office—including your computer administrator—don't evaluate the suggestions (and possibly complaints) of your personnel, you're closing a very valuable door.

Planning and Scheduling Computer Work

The organization of the work to be performed on the computer requires input from both you and your staff—and thoughtful planning. Some computer procedures should be scheduled on a daily basis, others weekly or monthly. The needs of your practice and any restrictions imposed by your software will help determine the work organization and schedules.

ACCOUNTS RECEIVABLE. All account information must be kept current. This responsibility must be assigned primarily to one individual (or, in larger practices, possibly two). She must be responsible for entering all changes involving accounts, such as change of address or any new information affecting a patient's third-party coverage. This updating should be done daily.

BANK DEPOSITS. A typical day of computer processing usually includes new-patient registration; the entering of data for charges, payments, and adjustments; and file maintenance. If the program allows for a daily bank-deposit record, it should total all daily deposits. If your software does not perform this function, the bank deposit should be prepared manually and its total compared to the total of the computer-processed payments. They must match; if they don't, the error must be found. By matching the totals on a daily basis, however, fewer errors will be made, and those that occur will be easier to find.

CHARTING A WORK SCHEDULE. Complete outlines should be charted for all data-processing functions: generation of insurance claims, statements, reports, other financial information, and so on. The work schedule should indicate when work is to be done and who is to do it. You can set it up on a daily, weekly, monthly, or even annual basis—although your best bet is probably to stick to a fairly short schedule—

daily or weekly. This schedule will supplement the job descriptions; it will reinforce each employee's understanding of the full extent of her responsibilities.

HANDLING DELAYS. But having a chart won't guarantee a smoothly running practice. The computer processing may not always be on schedule. Information that should be handled on a daily basis may get backed up. If this happens, the computer administrator needs to know why. Perhaps the physicians are simply not completing their portion of the service charge sheets. Or possibly the sheets aren't being forwarded properly to the business office. Problems of this sort are easily remedied, and they should not be ignored—or they'll help defeat the benefits gained through data processing. Only through the cooperation of everyone—physicians and staff—can all the potential benefits of a computer system be realized.

Keep in mind that most of your problems won't occur in the actual data processing, but will result from shortcomings in office organization or management control. When this becomes apparent, a specific plan of action should be developed to eliminate the problems and maintain control of the office operations.

Restricting Information, Access, and Functions

The computer administrator should make sure that all essential information relating to the computer system is on hand. The vendor should have provided manuals for the operation and application of all software. Instructional material should also be available on such functions as cleaning the printer and changing the ribbons and paper. This sort of information should always be readily accessible to your staff. (That doesn't mean, however, that you can't keep copies in a safe or fireproof cabinet in your office.) But while some information should be available to everyone, other information should be restricted, by a "need-to-know" kind of approach.

CHANGING PATIENT ACCOUNT NUMBERS. For example, you may occasionally want to change an account number—perhaps a patient has just been divorced, or just reached 21. Or it may be necessary to assign a new number because of the way your system is set up. If cycle billing is done by financial classification and a patient changes primary insurance carrier, a new number may be needed. But account numbers shouldn't be changed at random.

You must always know the reason an account number has been changed. That's reason enough to restrict this function to one individual—so you'll always know who made the change; so you can easily follow it up.

PURGING ACCOUNTS. Purging accounts is another function that should be restricted to as few individuals as possible. You'll probably want to start purging after you've had your computer for a while. After all, your disk space is limited, and it makes sense to remove any unnecessary data. So you may order that all zero-balance accounts inactive for a specified time be purged from the system to allow for new accounts. But the problem here is obvious: Anyone who can purge accounts could also knock out current accounts. A good share of accounts receivable could be wiped out with a keystroke.

Some programs, however, will allow purging only of zero-balance accounts inactive since some date you can specify. Other programs may allow for automatic purging by transaction date alone. Sometimes with this second type of program, transactions are purged even with outstanding balances. (The balances are not removed from the accounts receivable, but the supporting transactions are gone.) It's evident that you must understand fully the procedures and implications regarding purging accounts and transactions. Other media (hard-copy printout, microfilm, etc.) should always be used to store records of purged information.

WHAT EVERYONE MUST KNOW. While certain instructions should be made available only to a few people, others should be posted in the data-processing area for all to see: for example, where to call when there's a hardware or software problem and the computer administrator isn't available; who is responsible for backing up the system; and how to put the system back in operation after a power failure or other cause of downtime. You may also want to acquire additional manuals for your employees to supplement the standard ones.

MANAGE OR BE MANAGED. As previously stated, management and control of a computer system are not built into the system but must come from resources found within your office. But have you noticed that more and more vendors are offering management services? Of course, it's not without cost! In addition, more advertising is appearing for purchasing the physicians' accounts receivable.

Your objective is to make the computer work for you. If you're content with the system doing your accounting, insurance claim processing, and billing, you'll probably encounter many problems and need to seek outside help. The work being accomplished by the computer is not being managed properly.

Business management is a specialized field, and medical practice management consultants can provide the expertise you'll need for making your system work for you. But their skills will not eliminate the need for internal management and control of the business operations on a day-to-day basis.

Repairs and Maintenance

Adequate support and maintenance of your computer system are essential to your business operations. Downtime may be caused by special computer work; that is, the temporary work being done may prevent simultaneous data entry. Or downtime may be caused by mechanical failures. After all, the computer is a machine—and a very sophisticated one. A system may shut down completely, for example, if the printer breaks down. Obviously, downtime must be kept to a minimum for the most efficient operation.

SERVICE CONTRACTS. Service contracts may give you a false sense of security. Your main concern should be how quickly your call will bring a serviceman. You don't want to hear something like: "We'll be there as quickly as possible. There are only two calls ahead of you."

Those two calls might take all day; meanwhile, you're stuck with a system that's not operating.

Verbal promises don't mean anything. Get everything in writing. Know exactly what you're paying for and how soon you can expect hardware problems to be corrected. Some contracts guarantee that your system will not be permitted to remain down longer than a given number of hours without immediate attention by a technician.

HARDWARE AND SOFTWARE PROBLEMS. Hardware problems are usually corrected easily; most of these are relatively simple mechanical malfunctions. Software problems *may* sometimes be simple: for example, you've tried to get more out of a program than you can—you're overstepping its boundaries, exceeding available space. But software problems are often more complicated than typical hardware problems. Some or all of a particular program may need to be rewritten.

Fortunately, more stories are told about downtime than are actually experienced. Many new programs, though, will have bugs that need to be eliminated. Your system may have to be down while a critical program is being debugged.

HELP FROM YOUR VENDOR. Dealing with reliable vendors is the best way to be sure of competent and prompt help in dealing with problems. Some vendors will work hand-in-glove with the computer administrator so that on-site visits can be avoided for all but the toughest problems. They will make special efforts to teach the computer administrator what can go wrong—and how it can be fixed. Some vendors provide a diagnostic system via telephone modem. When a problem occurs, you hook into diagnostic equipment at the vendor's location. A service call can often be avoided when the problem is diagnosed and solved this way.

KEEPING UP WHEN THE COMPUTER IS DOWN. When downtime does occur, your personnel will have to carry on as usual. All necessary information should be compiled and saved to be entered when the computer is up again.

When the computer is down for a significant period of time, it will be necessary to rely on hard copy. The longer the system is down, the more difficult the problem becomes. But a competent computer administrator or office manager can keep the office running smoothly. And when downtime occurs—as it will—you'll acutely realize more than ever just how important the computer has become to your office.

21. What the Future Holds for You and Your Computer

Once you have your computer system in full operation, you can start thinking about your future needs—and wants. You may wish to begin immediately to incorporate other programs into your system. But don't rush into it. That should be a gradual process.

Justifying System Expansion

Just as you cost-justified (Chapter 3) the original purchase of your computer, you should also justify the purchase of any additional hardware or software. Before implementing any additional programs, evaluate your current system and the future goals of your practice. It's important to distinguish the current evaluation from the future projections; your needs could change quickly if, for example, you take on a new partner.

Planning is just as vital to the medical practice as it is to any business enterprise. Ask yourself: "What will my practice be like a year from now?" "Five years from now?" "Ten years from now?" Then ask yourself: "Will I be ready?"

Assume you do get a new partner and also hire an additional medical assistant. Previously, you might not have thought that a sophisticated computer accounting system was necessary. But with an additional partner and employee, you may find that a general ledger program (Chapter 18) is well worth the money.

When you're doing your cost-justification analysis for this or any other program, don't forget the support and maintenance costs vital to any program's success. Keep in mind, too, that your computer operators have to be trained for each new program you acquire.

Upgrading Your Computer's Accounting Capabilities

Your present computer accounting system may consist of an accounts-receivable program, which is fine for performing your main account-ing function—keeping track of income. But a general ledger program will also provide you with accounts-payable functions.

ACCOUNTS-PAYABLE PROGRAM. With this program, checks can be computer-generated. Daily payments and/or bank deposits can be posted into the system. And a general ledger program provides audit trails of all transactions.

Payroll checks can also be computer-generated. Tax computations for FICA, federal and state tax withholding, and any other money with-held from employees' pay will be handled by the computer.

OTHER FUNCTIONS. The general ledger program can provide a vari-ety of other useful functions, such as keeping track of depreciation schedules, generating complete income and expense records and quarterly and year-end reports, and filling out IRS-required income report forms. These are all discussed in more detail in Chapter 18 along with the methods for determining if this package is for you.

Your Continuing Involvement

Having some experience with a computer system doesn't eliminate management's responsibilities. To upgrade computer systems or pro-grams or to add new programs will require the same conscientious management effort the initial computerization did. Without your *con-tinuing* leadership role, it will be difficult for you to achieve current objectives, much less long-term ones.

You must plan ahead for *all* the activities that will be vital to the success of any new addition to your system. Specific duties to be performed must be categorized and assigned. If the computer operator does not know how to acquire the new input data needed, then you're not prepared to institute a new program.

The choice of data to be entered should enhance the overall operation. There should also be an established office organizational pattern to enable that data to flow smoothly and regularly to the personnel responsible for computer input.

In a small group practice, the computer administrator may be able to plan, organize, direct, and control the implementation of a new program. In a larger group, the computer administrator may be responsible for operating the computer system as efficiently as possible under your closer supervision. In either case, *your* interest and support (and that of the other physicians in the group) will be a major factor in the computer system's success.

Clinical Computer Applications

Of particular concern to you may be the medically oriented uses of the computer. While business programs for computers will probably be somewhat enhanced in the future, the state of the art is already quite advanced. Unfortunately, the same can't be said for clinical programs.

TODAY'S CLINICAL SOFTWARE. Most clinical computer programs in medical offices today aren't very sophisticated. For example, there are programs to assist with patient histories and physicals. They are designed to receive input on medical conditions, findings, and/or treatment. But some of these programs aren't much more than electronic filing systems, providing, perhaps, only the addition of patient-recall functions. The operator enters the date the patient is due to return for follow-up care, and the computer generates an appropriate and timely reminder.

More complex programs generate suggestions for medical management, based on the patient's history and findings. And patient information sheets can be computer-generated, summarizing your customary instructions regarding specific diagnoses, procedures, tests, or medications.

Automation is playing a substantial and beneficial role in medicine. But good programs in this area are difficult to write. For example, consider a program to assist in diagnosis: There are 750 different disease entities in internal medicine. Each has an average of 125 signs, symptoms, and laboratory findings. Figuring in the frequency of each disease, the computer can attempt to pick the most likely diagnoses, based on all the facts it is given about a specific patient.

When you multiply 750 by 125, then calculate in the frequency factor, you can see the massive amount of information the computer requires to assist in faster diagnosis of both complicated and run-of-the-mill cases.

Another task for medical software is to sift out problem cases. As one well-known cardiologist (whose practice is fully computerized) explains: "Most cases that are unusual aren't recognized as unusual. So we need to look at populations of patients and identify those who either are not responding to treatment or match a pattern that makes them special problems." A clinical program may allow you the capability to look at whole populations of patients with headaches, to find those who aren't responding well and who may have, say, brain tumors.

Clinical software is easily accessible by telephone from a national data base. In the near future, more doctors will probably have their own data base since storage (disk space) is becoming less costly.

Clinical software is overcoming at least two human shortcomings: First, our frail memories. We all have limited memories, and no one can retain the full knowledge base of medicine anymore. Second, our difficulty in decision making. As you well know, there are many tenable hypotheses in a typical diagnosis. And the rarer a diagnosis is, the less likely a physician is to think of it. A computer will help.

IS IT A THREAT? Some doctors see the notion of computers moving into diagnostic medicine as a threat. But remember that the physician will still make the final judgments. As one physician well versed in computers says: "Most of what I see in medicine is a combination of diagnosis *and* judgment. And when it comes to combining the two, the computer will always lose. The doctor will still be the decision-maker. Nothing will change except that computers will greatly expand his capacity to make sound decisions."

In sum, the next few years should see computers not only helping doctors administratively but also helping to decide why Mrs. Smith has a stomachache. The ultimate impact of computer technology in medicine will, no doubt, be determined by how we use it.

A Final Word

As you gradually incorporate new programs into your system, time must be allowed for training of key personnel. Although courses are available, the real training occurs right in your office after the program has been implemented. This holds true both for the more sophisticated business programs now available and for tomorrow's clinical software.

Once you have your team assembled and your plan mapped out, you're ready to plunge into the future. There will always be periods of trial and error, but don't get discouraged. If you really want computerization to work—and you're willing to make the personal commitment—it will work. And when it does, the rewards will be huge.

Glossary
of Computer Terms

ANSI. American National Standards Institute, an organization that develops data-processing standards that are widely used as guidelines in the industry.

applications programs. Programs designed to provide specific functions for the user; user input is usually necessary to run these programs. See systems programs.

ASCII. American Standard Code for Information Interchange, an 8-bit code for internal computer representation of up to 128 characters.

assembler. See translator.

assembly language. A machine-oriented programming language. Each assembly language instruction corresponds to a single machine instruction.

audit trail. A record of all the events relating to a transaction, from initial entries through final report. In a computer system, the trail is created during the routine processing of data, allowing system audits or reconstruction of lost transactions.

backup. Provision for alternative means of operation in case of primary failure; a copy preserved, often on a different medium, as a safeguard against destruction of original data or processed information; any resource needed for disaster recovery.

BASIC. Acronym for "Beginner's All-purpose Symbolic Instruction Code," a computer language designed to be easy for neophytes to master.

batch processing. A procedure in which an accumulation of items (such as transactions) is grouped for eventual processing as a single unit. See on-line processing.

baud. A unit of measure of data flow speed; one signal element (usually one bit) per second.

benchmark program. A sample program used to test and compare the performance of different computers.

binary notation. Representation of numeric values in the base 2 number system, using only 0s and 1s. Computers use base 2 numbers internally because two states (such as on and off) are easily implemented.

bit. A binary digit; a 0 or 1; hence, a unit of information in binary notation.

black box. An unspecified device or process that performs a specific function, or in which known inputs produce known outputs in a fixed relationship.

bootstrapping. Starting up of an inoperative system by an automatic subroutine whose first instructions call the rest of itself into the computer; invoked from the console.

branch. A departure from the straight-line sequence in a program, caused by a conditional or unconditional branch instruction; also called jump.

bug. An error in a computer program; occasionally also used to refer to a hardware defect.

bus. A circuit or path over which data are transmitted.

byte. A sequence of adjacent bits considered as a unit; almost always synonymous with 8-bit byte, equivalent to one character.

canned software. See package, software.

cathode-ray tube (CRT). An electronic vacuum tube in which a beam of electrons can be focused to produce a visible display on a video screen.

central processing unit (CPU). The computer's main unit and nerve center; it contains the circuits that execute instructions.

character. An elementary symbol belonging to a set. The usual set of characters the computer can read, store, and write includes decimal digits 0–9, letters A–Z, punctuation marks, and operation symbols.

chip. An integrated circuit or circuits on a (usually silicon) wafer slice; the basis for the microcomputer.

COBOL. Acronym for "COmmon Business Oriented Language," a computer language designed for general commercial data processing and widely used in industry.

compiler. See translator.

computer language. A defined set of characters, symbols, words, etc., and the rules for combining them into meaningful communications for conveying instructions or data to the computer. See assembly language; high-level language; machine language.

console. The computer operator's control panel for communicating with the computer; the console has control keys, display lights, and a keyboard; it enables the operator to control the machine manually.

core memory. A term originally applied to a configuration of ferrite cores, capable of holding a magnetic polarization, used for main memory storage. This technology has largely been replaced by semiconductor memory, but the term has been generalized to refer to any main memory—the memory component of the CPU and the computer's fastest storage device.

CPU. Central processing unit.

crash. A breakdown or failure resulting in downtime.

CRT. Cathode-ray tube.

CRT terminal. An input/output device basically consisting of a video screen, control unit, and keyboard.

cursor. A moving position indicator on a video screen display indicating where data may be entered or a correction made.

data. Basic elements of information that can be processed or produced by a computer.

data base. A usually large and continuously updated file of information on a particular subject or subjects; designed for easy search and retrieval.

debugging. The process of detecting, diagnosing, and correcting errors in computer programs; occasionally also refers to correcting hardware flaws.

disk drive. The magnetic disk's power unit.

diskette. A small magnetic disk made of flexible Mylar material; also known as floppy disk.

disk, magnetic. A random-access mass storage device consisting of a circular metal plate that continuously rotates as it is accessed by a read/write head. Disks may be permanently mounted or removable.

disk pack. A stack of disk platters enclosed in a case, designed to be placed in a processing device and used as a single unit.

distributed data processing. Use of more than one computer in geographically dispersed locations to perform related tasks in a cooperative manner.

documentation. All documents, manuals, diagrams, etc., associated with a computer system. *Program* documentation is used to supplement the language code, explaining program design and purposes.

downtime. Any period during which a computer (or other device) is unavailable for use. This may be due to breakdown, malfunction, repair time, or maintenance.

EBCDIC. Expanded Binary-Coded Decimal Interchange Code, an 8-bit code for internal computer representation of up to 256 characters; used especially on IBM systems.

edit. To format data for subsequent processing; to make changes in a file involving insertions, deletions, transpositions, or corrections.

EDP. Electronic data processing.

field. A subdivision of a record containing a unit of information. Examples: name field and Social Security number field in a payroll record.

file. A group of related records, usually residing on magnetic disk or tape, treated as a unit. A file can contain data, programs, or both, and is addressed by a file name.

file maintenance. Modification of file contents to correct errors; distinguished from *updating*—changes made in a file to reflect real changes in the events recorded in the file.

firmware. A cross between hardware and software; computer programs hard-wired (physically embodied) in the hardware.

floppy disk. See diskette.

FORTRAN. Acronym for "FORmula TRANslation," a computer language designed for scientific and mathematical use, but now widely used for commercial applications, as well.

GIGO. Acronym for "Garbage In, Garbage Out," expressing the principle that unreliable input data produce unreliable output data.

hard copy. A printed copy of computer output in a visually readable and permanent form.

hardware. Physical components of a computer system. See software.

header. A set of identifying and other types of data appearing in a defined format at the beginning of a file.

high-level language. A computer programming language that is relatively independent of the limitations of any specific computer. A program written in a high-level language must go through a translation process before it can be executed by a computer. Examples: BASIC, COBOL, FORTRAN, Pascal.

input. To enter information into the computer; information so entered.

intelligent terminal. A terminal containing logic circuits in its hardware, enabling it to handle some limited processing of data on its own, independently of the processor to which it is connected.

interactive system. A system placing the user in direct, "conversational" communication with the computer, providing immediate response to user input.

interface. A common boundary between two devices, systems, or processes; the point where independent systems or processes communicate or interact.

interpreter. See translator.

JCL. Job control language, codes for issuing requests to the operating system regarding the processing of jobs.

K. An abbreviation for kilo, or thousand; in computer parlance, because of the binary nature of computers, 1K equals 1,024, the nearest power of 2 to 1,000.

load. To enter programs or data into core memory.

loop. A series of program instructions executed repeatedly until some terminal condition is satisfied.

lpm. Lines per minute; used to describe output speed of a line printer.

machine language. A code expressing instructions that can be read and used directly by the computer without further processing or translation.

mainframes. The largest computers, essentially distinguished from the minicomputer category by relative price, size, speed of execution, and computing power.

main memory. See core memory.

mass storage. A peripheral device directly addressable by the CPU, with a large memory capacity compared with main memory; same as secondary storage. Examples: magnetic tape, disk.

mega-. Million; e.g., 1 megabyte equals 1 million bytes.

memory. A device that can store information for later retrieval; same as storage.

menu. A terminal display of a list of optional facilities that can be chosen by the user to perform various functions.

microcomputer. The smallest of computers; its CPU consists of semiconductor integrated circuits. Desktop personal computers fall into this category.

minicomputer. A computer usually larger, more expensive, and more powerful than a microcomputer; less powerful and versatile than a mainframe.

modem. Acronym for "MOdulator DEModulator," a device that converts data from a form compatible with computer equipment to a form compatible with transmission facilities (such as telephone lines), and vice versa.

multiprocessing. Use of multiple computers in tandem, sharing input/output devices; two or more processors (one in control, others subordinate) in a system configuration.

multiprogramming. A computer system's ability to handle a number of programs concurrently by interleaving their execution.

object code (program). A sequence of code in binary form, resulting from conversion of source code by a translator, which is ready for computer execution. Most software packages supply only object code.

off line. Independent; not under direct control of the CPU.

on line. Under direct control of the CPU.

on-line processing. A procedure in which each transaction or data unit is processed immediately as it becomes available to the processor. See batch processing.

operating system. A software package, usually provided by the equipment manufacturer, designed to control the computer's basic resources. The operating system handles such tasks as scheduling, loading, and running of applications programs; controlling input and output devices; and managing spooling, multiprogramming, and core memory.

output. The generation of information by the computer; the information so generated.

package, software. A generalized program written for a major application, designed to be useful to a wide range of users; also called prepackaged software; canned software.

parallel processing. Simultaneous operation of an old and new system so the results produced by the new system may be compared for accuracy with those produced by the old.

Pascal. A highly structured computer language designed to enhance the teaching of programming as a systematic discipline; named for 17th-century mathematician Blaise Pascal.

password. A unique and confidential set of characters and/or digits to be typed on a terminal keyboard, by which a user identifies himself to the computer system. The system will grant the user a defined level of information access based on his password.

patch. A set of instructions inserted into a program to change, update, or correct it.

peripheral device. A physically separate input, output, or storage device operated under computer control. Examples: printer, disk drive, magnetic tape drive, CRT terminal.

power supply, uninterruptible. Backup battery power to enable continuous operation of a computer system during power failures.

printer. An electromechanical device that expresses output data as printed hard copy.

printer, line. A printing device that prints an entire line at a time.

printer, matrix. A printing device that prints a character at a time in character-like configurations of dots.

processor. Usually synonymous with CPU.

program. A set of instructions or steps directing a computer to perform a specific function.

programming language. See computer language.

queue. A line or collection of items waiting for the attention of the processor or a peripheral device.

RAM. Random-access memory.

random-access memory (RAM). A type of storage providing immediate access to any memory location.

read. The copying of data from one form of storage to another; particularly from external or secondary storage to internal storage. See write.

read-only memory (ROM). A device storing information that can be read, but not changed.

real-time system. Any system that processes input data virtually simultaneously with the event generating the data.

reasonableness check. Test of input data to ensure it falls within an expected range, an attempt to detect errors; also called validity check.

record. A unit of data made up of a set of one or more fields; a basic element of a file. Example: an employee's payroll record.

remote job entry (RJE). Entry of computer programs and data into a remote terminal for transmission to the central processor.

RJE. Remote job entry.

ROM. Read-only memory.

routine. A program or program segment; a software procedure that performs some well-defined function.

secondary storage. See mass storage.

semiconductor memory. Memory using active transistor circuits as memory cells, capable of storing information as one of two (binary) states.

sequential storage. A device requiring data to be accessed only in the sequence in which it was stored; also called serial storage.

serial storage. See sequential storage.

service bureau. A company supplying access to off-premises computer services; users supply input data and pay for the results.

software. All the programs that can be used on a particular computer system. See hardware; package, software.

sorting. Arranging (ordering) data items according to some predefined rules of sequence using a key, or preselected field, contained in each item.

source code (program). The original high-level-language version of a computer program, requiring conversion by a language translator before it can be executed by a computer; usually not included in a software package. See object code.

source document. A document supplying basic data to be entered into the computer system.

spooling. A term originally derived from SPOOL, an acronym for "Simultaneous Peripheral Output On Line," now extended to refer to input, as well. Spooling is a software feature by which input from or output to slow devices is placed into queues on mass storage to await transmission.

storage. See memory.

subroutine. A self-contained section of a program that performs a logical function contributing to the program's overall purpose. It can be invoked repeatedly from anywhere in the main program.

system. The computer hardware, software, and all related components.

systems analyst. A systems designer; one who analyzes user requirements and develops them into a conceptual framework.

systems programs. Programs constituting the computer's operating system, designed to provide basic system functions such as input, output, and job scheduling. See applications programs.

tape drive. The magnetic tape's power unit.

tape, magnetic. A sequential or serial mass storage device consisting of a continuous ribbon of magnetic-coated material wound on a reel.

terminal. A computer input/output device; often used synonymously with CRT terminal.

throughput. Productivity of a system based on all facets of its operation, expressed in transaction volume or speed; a measure of processing power.

time sharing. Use of a device for two or more purposes concurrently.

transaction. A set of related exchanges between a terminal user and a computer system.

translator. A program that converts a sequence of statements in one language or coding system to an equivalent sequence of statements in another. Compilers, assemblers, and interpreters are types of translators.

turnkey system. A complete computer system for which a single vendor assumes total responsibility for hardware and software construction, installation, and testing.

user-friendly. Designed with an emphasis on the user's point of view; assisting the user and making his task as easy and understandable as possible.

utilities. "Housekeeping" programs; standard routines supplied with a computer system. Examples: diagnostic, sorting, file-manipulation, directory-listing, and debugging routines.

validity check. See reasonableness check.

VDT. Visual display terminal.

video screen. Screen attached to input/output equipment designed for visual display.

visual display terminal (VDT). Any device permitting computer input by keyboard or other manual means and output by visual display on a CRT.

word. A basic unit of data in computer memory; a predetermined number of bits treated as an entity; often a multiple of byte length.

word processing. A set of automated operations to aid in producing letter-quality documents. These include text editing, formatting, storage and retrieval of a library of form letters, pagination, and printing of the final draft.

write. The copying of data to an output medium, usually from internal storage to external storage. See read.

Index